$1.00

MW00893507

One Size Fits All Diet

My Story of Survival

FIVE YEARS ON TEN INGREDIENTS ONLY

FOR BREAKFAST LUNCH AND DINNER
EVERY SINGLE DAY

Add oodles of faith

A true story

Ultimate low reactive diet for allergies, gut problems,
food intolerances and chemical sensitivities

---

by M Emmanuel

My Story of Survival – One Size Fits All Diet (OSFA)
five years on ten ingredients only

is dedicated to those seeking health.

first edition 2014 - second edition March 2015 – November 2015

ISBN-13: 978-1522734895

DISCLAIMER - This book nor the author seeks to diagnose or treat illness or give advice to anyone seeking treatment for any kind of health condition. Anyone reading the information in this book should take this account as a personal story, which the author is sharing with the intention of inspiring other seekers in collaboration with their own medical professional health advisor to come up with their own solutions. The author is not a medical professional and has no qualifications as a licensed medical expert. Readers should not rely on the information in this book for any reason whatsoever, but should instead consult with their medical practitioner and rely on the licensed health practitioner's advice before engaging in a health program or starting a new diet. The author is not affiliated with any organisation as noted in this book unless this is specifically mentioned.

Another Mosaic House publication.
The author can be contacted at www.mosaichouse.co
PB 25 Noosa, Qld 4567, Australia
All rights reserved – ©2015 myemmanuel. The content, formatting and design may not in any way be emulated, reproduced, duplicated or copied in any manner without prior written permission from the publisher.

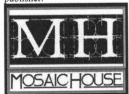

Created in the Commonwealth of Australia
Printed and distributed in the United States of America

Cover design by Nehara of creativelog
Formatting by SunnyEdesign

THANK YOU!

Thank you for <u>leaving a review on Amazon</u> if you feel that you benefited from reading my story. Your review will help other readers find my book and reviews show me that all the hard work was not in vain. Below are some reviews about My Story of Survival from Amazon Readers.

Amazon Reviews

<u>I highly recommend this well written</u> ...

I can relate to Ms. Emmanuel's story of survival. I'm deeply grateful to her for writing this book. My wife has a history of similar experiences. Her appendix ruptured leading to a cascade of health issues. We've seen dozens of doctors all over the US, and gotten many diagnoses. Yet none of them lead to effective treatment. As a medical professional myself I know the tremendous impact of diet on health. My wife has shown significant improvement over the past 2 years after embarking on a vegan diet. I think a modified version of Ms. Emmanuel's plan may help get to yet another level of recovery. It's certainly worth a try. I highly recommend this well written, easily relatable work. It is a real blessing. N. Clark, December 14, 2015

<u>An amazing true story</u>

An amazing true story! Love how Mimi's writing style is very down to earth and makes it feel as if she's sitting in your living room telling her story. I enjoyed the 'little extra facts' sprinkled throughout the chapters. Seeing her faith in God weaved so seamlessly in her life was encouraging as well. Amazon Customer, December 17, 2015

<u>Inspirational True Story Of Love, Faith and Courage Through Life Threatening Food Intolerance.</u>

My Story of Survival: Five years on ten ingredients only, ultimate low reactive diet by Mimi Emmanuel is a book of courage, love and faith and not necessarily a diet book. The author went through years of the inability to tolerate any foods and faced near death experiences on several occasions. Through the help of family and friends and some open-minded health practitioners, she used exclusion, slowly trying different foods she could tolerate. If not for her family and her own tenacity and faith, she would not have lived. This is a story that is compelling and touching. The author had to go for over five years eating just ten ingredients that she could tolerate and small amounts of those at that. I recommend this book to anyone who has trouble with tolerating the chemical saturated and genetically engineered foods we are eating, as well as over-prescribed medications, or anyone who likes a good true story of courage, faith and determination. Although she doesn't advocate the usage of her own diet, it is, at least a starting point for anyone suffering from similar problems. David A Dill, December 22, 2015

Amazing personal story of surviving incredible food allergies and health issues!

I was blown away by this story. I didn't even realize it was possible to live on only 10 ingredients, much less for 5 years! Mimi's story is filled with faith and hope. I found myself so anxious tor her success as I read through her process. Thankfully, I do not suffer from food allergies, but found inspiration going far beyond just Mimi finding a menu that worked for her. The faith and confidence in God that she expresses is inspiring for anyone going through tough times. Tiffany H. Allen, December 17, 2015

This book may save someone's life

Emmanuel has written a guide that I think can save someones life in the future. She writes of the ingredients that are the safest to take in our bodies. It's well written, and as I was reading it, I couldn't help but feel the writer's pain and struggles. Even though I, personally, don't suffer from anything (though after reading this, who knows...we all may have just a little something), I think the book is a great resource for anyone suffering from "random" food intolerance ... Highly recommended for those who are looking for something---anything---to fix their body problems. Mark Bacera, December 16, 2015

This is a God-send read for those with mysterious food intolerance.

At the end of your digestive rope? Hang on, you are not alone and have a friend who can help! This is an honest-to-goodness real story of one woman's grit and self-determination when faced with an over-whelming medical conundrum as to why her body was on revolt.

You can't be the master of a sinking ship without becoming a master builder; becoming a student on how to patch and re-build. Mimi Emmanuel learned how to craft her own survival diet out of just a very few ingredients. While she hopes that none of her readers would ever have to follow her diet, she shares this journey to show that there are answers to be found. There are times when the standard elimination diet is far too broad for those suffering from a fried immune and digestive system.

She shares the spartan but nourishing diet she had to follow for FIVE years as well as how she has tippy-toed into a more varied Phase 2. I especially like her "useful facts" that she places throughout the book to not only make her case as to nutritional needs, but they also spark a deeper interest for further study and personal application. I will most definitely recommend this book to those I teach about diet and nutrition. Deidre J. Edwards, December 6, 2015

The digital version of 'My Story of Survival' launched on Amazon at 6pm AEST on December 15, 2015 and that very moment our internet was interrupted for the whole duration of the launch free-promo-period (a full three days). Despite this major interruption, which meant that I was not able in any way to promote my book or even be at my own 'online' launch party, only days after its launch, 'My Story of Survival' ranked among Amazon's Bestsellers in the categories of Nutrition and Medical ebooks, #1 Food Allergies, #1 Digestive Organs, #1 Irritable bowel, #1 in Chronic Pain, #1 Science, #1 Viral and #2 Health, Diet and Fitness Short Reads. It also received the bestsellers badge under Catholicism/self-help.

None of this would have occurred if not for the support of my fellow students and my Friends from Above. THANK YOU!!

Thank you for purchasing my book. If you would like to receive a free Kindle of my next book, you can indicate so by visiting www.mosaichouse.co/my-story-of-survival and I will contact you when the next promotion is on so that you can download a free Kindle of my next ebook.

TABLE OF CONTENTS

DEDICATION

This book, 'My Story of Survival,' which presents a One Size Fits All (OSFA) diet plan, is dedicated to all of us who need a little help balancing our meals with our health requirements and to all the angels that kept me going.

FOREWORD

I've asked Greg Turner to write the foreword for my One Size Fits All (OSFA) diet plan, simply because I think that he possibly does not agree with this diet plan, and I figure that he can write a decent counter balance foreword without tearing my diet to shreds. He also, alongside my children, pulled out all the stops to keep me going after I ruptured my appendix. Greg really knows his stuff. Lifesaving diet, really? It may not be for others, but it was for me.

Writing this foreword to Mimi Emmanuel's little book has been challenging to me personally, as I felt I could not possibly endorse the concept of eating only ten foods to obtain all the nutrients necessary for sustaining life.

The very idea goes against everything taught at university about nutrition and its relation to wellness.

However, since I first met Mimi some six years ago, I have witnessed how she has slowly started to regain her health through a process that could be described as an experiment in   survival.

Mimi's illness is primarily about food chemical sensitivity.

Many people know, for instance, that they react to MSG or metabisulphite in food and drink, and assiduously avoid these where possible to avoid the nasty effects.

3

Mimi, however, reacts to naturally-occurring constituents in common foods as well as the plethora of additives, preservatives, flavours, colours, and extracts which the food industry insists we need in our foods to make them saleable products.

If we add in pesticide and herbicide residues in vegetables, fruits, grains, and meats, then the extent of chemical soup in our lives becomes more clear.

Illness relating to fatigue, debility, and muscle pain are testament to a food chain becoming increasingly more toxic.

A diet containing organically-grown food is of the utmost importance to assist recovery from these serious debilitating illnesses.

So we have Mimi's OSFA diet, perhaps the ultimate low-reactive diet plan. It may be a good place to start when no other answers seem forthcoming, although I advise caution, as it is vital to try to get as diverse a range of foods in your diet as possible.

Perhaps Mimi could have called it The "It Worked For Me Diet."

Gregory Turner N.D. Grad. Dip. Health Science (Nutrition Medicine).

4

INTRO

Another diet book, nooo!!! However, this book is different, very different. Why? This book is unlike any other cook or diet book because the whole book only has ten main ingredients in it. And that's for breakfast, lunch, and dinner.
Ha! Told you that this book is different, didn't I?

The first edition of this book I wrote for my family. The second edition was to be shared freely to help others who are struggling with their health. With this third edition, I am filling in some gaps with my testimony. Every breath I take I owe to my Creator, and every step I take is dedicated to Him. I am sharing my story because I know that others will benefit from it. My ten-ingredients-only diet played a large and important part in my recovery, but it was not the only part, nor was it the most important part that helped me recover.

The most important part of my recovery was and still is my faith and the help I received from up High. I am head over heels with the Author of my favourite Book and I am learning to follow his guidance in my life and accept his nudges and prompts; so far with excellent results.

I'm still here, yeah!! And sharing with you, too good!
I've decided to publish this third edition on Amazon so that more people have access to it.
If one person only will be helped from hearing my story, then it was worth writing it down.

Don't follow me!

This diet plan is not only different because it has only ten ingredients in it, but it is also different because I don't expect anyone who reads the menu to actually follow the list of options mentioned. No doubt you're now thinking that this book is perhaps a con? Well, it's far from it. It's my own personal story; it is documenting a tiny part of my fight back to health.

The reason that this book only has ten main ingredients in it is because that is about all I can tolerate. I didn't purposely set out to eat ten ingredients only. At some stage, my health crumbled to the extent that ten ingredients in total was all I could tolerate without experiencing severe side effects. And the reason that I don't think that anyone will follow it is because I doubt that anyone would be disciplined enough to only eat ten ingredients for all their meals unless they had no other choice. I like to think that most people are able to eat a much wider variety of foods.

To follow my diet for a short period of time, however, when no other answers are forthcoming, may be a life saver; as it certainly has been for me. The way Greg puts it, my One Size Fits All (OSFA) Diet may be the ultimate low-reactive diet plan. The OSFA Diet may be useful for people who are in need of a quick, temporary solution when they suffer from gut problems, chemical sensitivities, food intolerances, and allergies.

What does low reactive mean? A low-reactive diet plan means that the foods included in this plan are the least likely to cause any negative reaction.

A popular diet to follow for people who suffer from food

intolerances is the low FODMAP diet which was developed at Monash University in Melbourne by Peter Gibson and Susan Shepherd. I didn't know about this diet when I was experiencing gut problems and if I had known about it, I would not have been able to stick to this diet because there are many ingredients in the low FODMAP diet that I am not able to tolerate. I'm probably an extreme case. The reason I mention this diet here is because it may be a good choice for people who can adhere to the low FODMAP diet.

*** **USEFUL FACT** *** *The term FODMAP is an acronym, deriving from "Fermentable Oligo-, Di-, Mono-saccharides And Polyols." These carbohydrates are commonly found in the modern western diet. Some evidence has been presented that the restriction of these FODMAPs from the diet may have a beneficial effect for sufferers of irritable bowel syndrome and other functional gastrointestinal disorders (FGID). See NOTES.*

Rainbow-coloured diet

Did you know that carrots originally grew in various colours? Years ago we had purple, white, and yellow, as well as orange carrots. The greater variety of food we are able to eat, the greater the chances are that we are eating a well-balanced diet. In the past, I aimed to eat as many colours as possible in any one day; for instance, red tomato, orange pumpkin, yellow capsicum, green lettuce, blue berries, purple cabbage, white rice, and so on.

Apart from the visual appeal, all the colours in the various foods naturally contain a diverse set of nutrients and vitamins.

Before my health crashed spectacularly, I used to incorporate all the colours of the rainbow in our daily menu planning because this was an easy guide to wholesome diet planning. One day I may be able to get back to that. Meanwhile, however, I'm enjoying my ten ingredient diet or the One Size Fits All (OSFA) diet.

Prepare it anyway you like

This diet book is differs from other books and not only because: A) it has a mere ten ingredients in it, and B) I don't actually expect anyone to follow it in the same way that I have. This diet also differs from other diets because if anyone were to be interested in sampling the diet, they're welcome to prepare the ten ingredients in any way that they like. Mash them, puree, boil, whatever takes your fancy. The only parameters are that you're relaxed when you eat and fully enjoy your food.

Very different

As I said before, this diet really is very different from any diet you've ever come across. There are only three guidelines.

1. Ten ingredients
2. Prepare them any way you like
3. Be relaxed when you eat and enjoy the meal.

Ten ingredients only

So why am I sharing my ten ingredients with my readers? Because I know that there are many people out there who are struggling with their diet for many reasons. Family members and friends have shared with me their own up-and-down love affairs with a whole range of delectable foods.

It is hard to eliminate certain favourites from our diet, even when we know that these food substances constantly give us grief. It becomes near impossible to get back to base when we don't know which ingredients from the menu cause adverse reactions, or if nearly all ingredients we consume have an adverse effect. Or indeed, when the suggested elimination diet is so boring and unsatisfying that it is not practical or possible for most people to stick with.

I've lived on just ten ingredients for the last five years, so I know that it works. For some of the five years, I even lived on a mere seven or even less ingredients because I wasn't able to tolerate anything raw, such as snow peas, or sweet, such as apple or fig, or dairy, such as yoghurt. And even on the seven or less ingredients, I was making progress because the paramount issue at the time for me, with a fragile digestive system, was to eliminate anything that aggravated my digestive processes.

One size fits all (OSFA)?

As in, really? Yes, really. Because this diet will suit people with even the most wide-ranging food intolerances. And if this diet, as I followed it, doesn't do the trick, then it can be easily adjusted to do so.

How did this diet come about? It came about when we had to figure out what to do when I found myself unable to process most food substances without adverse effects.

No gluten, no dairy, no sugars, no flours, no meat, no nuts, no seeds, no eggs, no beans, no lentils, no soy, and no grains such as rice nor any other grain.

To be diagnosed gluten intolerant or a coeliac is bad enough. But, what if you also cannot tolerate gluten-free flours, dairy, soy, a whole range of vegetables and fruit, sugars, any kind of grain, nuts, seeds, beans, eggs, chicken, nor meat? Read on.

CHAPTER ONE
A LITTLE HISTORY

BURNOUT

In a nutshell, I burned out. Like, real good. I managed three medical clinics; my husband, who is a GP, worked in these clinics. I also took care of hubby, raised our children, kept the home, moved house a few times, never quite recovered properly from a bout of double pneumonia, got stressed, and then in my early forties whilst moving house once more and carrying oodles of boxes, began haemorrhaging and continued to do so for a number of weeks. By the time I finished moving house, I lost a massive amount of blood and ever since I have suffered from orthostatic intolerance.

Orthostatic intolerance is a fancy word for not being able to stand up straight for long periods of time. It's the same condition that the front man Greg Page from The Wiggles was diagnosed with, and what made him withdraw from the lucrative business of the Wiggles for a period of five years.

The main problem for me with this condition is that I didn't realise I had the condition, and as such, I continued to push through. I think that many people who work in the medical industry think that they are invincible, and I was certainly one of them. In the end, we all have our limits, and I only realised this long after I had pushed well and truly through all of them many times over. It is a really dumb thing to ignore one's physical and emotional limitations, and I paid a high price for doing so.

Eventually, as I limped along, I picked up the odd bug here and there, which I wasn't able to shrug off like I used to in the past.

From bad to worse

Whatever I did to compensate for working all hours wasn't working. Long story short, it went from bad to worse, and from living a healthy active life where I was able to eat anything I like, too bit-by-bit, becoming increasingly unable to tolerate various foods. I developed infections and chemical sensitivities and finally found myself mainly confined to bed. Only when I'm horizontal and supported, away from noise, light, movement and smells, is my body not suffering. At my worst I've been confined to bed in a darkened room without being able to say or do anything much at all, for months and months on end. The problem with this is of course that muscles need exercise and human beings need human interaction.

It took me quite a while to realise that I was not able to eat the way I used to, work the way I used to, exercise the way I used to, and socialise the way I used to. I used to work 24/7 under hugely stressful circumstances, and I believe that in the end, the ongoing stress is what conditioned me to ignore whatever was going on in my body.

Despite my best efforts, I had not been able to reduce many of the stresses I was under and I had gotten into the habit of ignoring whatever I was not able to solve. Applying the same technique to my health and wellbeing didn't get me the results I was after either.

The medical industry did what the medical industry does with various tests and diagnoses. I did what I did, joking around with family and friends, telling them that I was just lying about all day, enjoying life whilst at night the rivers of tears flowed freely. After a number of years, I signed up for a dodgy medical trial on the internet which was supposed to finally get me back on my feet.

The cocktails of antibiotics prescribed to me during the trial set me up for a number of pancreatic attacks. This was followed shortly after by an emergency hospital admission with an inoperable ruptured appendix with septicaemia. By then, probably as perks of the trial, I had developed intolerance to antibiotics.

Terrifying premonition

Just before we moved house in the year 2008, one of my daughters had a terrifying premonition, which came to her in a dream.

"Mum, it was one of those dreams where everything was crystal clear, just as I've had before, remember? And that dream came true too. It was terrifying; the doctor said to us 'there is a two in three chance she won't make it.' He was talking about you, Mum, and he meant it. It was serious."

At the time, all I could think to do was to calm my shaking and teary daughter, so I wiped her tears, looked her straight in the eyes and said, *"I promise to be careful darling. Don't you worry about a thing, God is in charge of us and our life is in his hands, always."*

It was less than two weeks after my daughter's 'nightmare' that the three of us found ourselves in the emergency

15

department with the surgeon telling my daughters that they wouldn't operate on me, fearing that my survival rate would be less than 2 in 5 if they did so.

The warning that had come to my daughter in her 'dream' was that, at the time my survival was at stake, I shouldn't take anything that would be offered to me. My daughter remembered and heeded this warning, which resulted in her refusing the morphine I was offered to cope with the relentless hurting of a ruptured appendix. Only after an abundance of prayer and a night of intolerable pain would my daughters yield and allow the nurse to give me a morphine injection.

I am now convinced that this may have saved my life because, considering the state I was in, I am pretty sure that a morphine shot would have allowed me to sink into blissful oblivion, never to return.

As it was, the hideous hurting kept me on edge and alert enough to want to stay around for my kids. I believe that if the inevitable relaxation that a morphine shot eventually did bring on had happened earlier, this potentially might have allowed the septicaemia to spread more than it did and cause more damage.

Prayers answered

Alleluia, Praise God, he heard our prayers, got me out of the hospital and into the care of my girls, who did an awesome job at keeping me going. It took the kids around a year to nurse me back to being able to simply get up from bed.

The hospital had sent me home with boxes of antibiotics to which I was intolerant, and with every breath I managed to take, I felt and looked as if it were going to be my last.

The surgeons had told me, *"Come back when you're better and we'll take your appendix out."*

The kids phoned around and located a wonderful naturopath who did a home visit and prescribed the homeopathic remedy Pyrogen and Cleavers herb. These remedies, together with loads of TLC and mustard seed-sized faith, proved to be a lifesaver.

When I came out of hospital mid-2008 after rupturing my appendix, I could only suck slivers of ice for quite a while. I couldn't drink, I couldn't eat, and there was nothing I could keep down, not even water, unless it had been frozen and shaved. The healthy diet I had been on of fresh, raw, organic vegs and fruit now caused me massive cramps and vomiting. After weeks, I was able to hold down some soups. After months passed, we discovered that I was unable to tolerate any kind of grain, including rice, or any kind of flour, meat, tofu, tempeh, cheeses (and I do like cheese), eggs, and so on. After a while, we figured out what I could tolerate, which we'll get to later.

Rest

So here we are now, some five years later. We decided to give my brave and courageous heart, pancreas, and appendix a rest. Why brave and courageous? Well, my heart faltered a couple of times. My appendix ruptured and my pancreas got attacked (by the antibiotics?) yet all showed me their fighting spirit, not giving up nor checking out, instead staying resolute and hanging in there. I feel that the least I can do is give my organs time out to relax and recuperate.

I wouldn't recommend that anyone eats only ten ingredients for years on end. But, it kept me going and, God willing, will keep me going whilst I continue to add in little bits and pieces at a time to come to a more varied and less restricted diet.

I didn't deliberately restrict my calorie intake but I found that practicing the art of laying about doesn't require a huge calorie intake. It also appears that having the right mineral balance doesn't just reduce cravings but completely obliterates them. More on that later when I mention my regular intake of sole (Himalayan salt brine).

*** **FUN FACT** *** *Taking in fewer calories slows metabolism, and some data indicate that humans with a slower metabolism live longer. Calorie restriction is pretty much the only thing out there that we know will not just prevent disease but also extend maximal life span. See NOTES.*

Genes

So what's the problem? The lectins in all the other foods? The lactose? The salicylates? The gluten? The sugars, the carbs, the oils?

Obviously, the food substances themselves aren't the problem because the majority of people seem to have no trouble with any of them. My responses, the food intolerances, are merely pointing to an underlying problem. There has to be an underlying health condition that causes the reactions I experience to most foods, chemicals, supplements, and the environment. The trick is to find out what this underlying health condition is.

As I'm writing this book, recent pathology tests have revealed certain genes that predispose people to certain things, such as in my case, re-occurring and persistent infections and the 'coeliac' gene.

Does this mean that when one has certain genes they also have certain conditions? No, it does not mean that. It means that the majority of people with certain conditions are found to have certain genes. For instance, the majority of people who have been diagnosed as a coeliac appear to have a particular gene.

However, there are people who have the same genes and don't suffer from the same symptoms. For the symptoms to manifest, one has to create the right environment first. Such as not scheduling rest, relaxation and proper sleep, which are all needed for a body to repair and stay in good nick.

Give the genes a helping hand

To get the symptoms of particular gene manifestations to blossom and kick in early in life, it is useful to have a collection of certain kinds of genes and get into the habit of skipping meals, eating dinner in 3 ½ minutes flat, handle whatever gets thrown at you without ever saying no; just practice being that super human who lives on air whilst moving mountains. Getting solidly grounded in those habits of testing your weaker genes to the max should yield positive results within a few years. It certainly worked for me.

I had to work at the crumbling of my empire for a few decades before it caved. When it caved, however, it did so spectacularly, with all the flickers and flashes my hard work deserved.

There is nothing wrong with gluten, milk and cheese, or sugar and lectins, and so on. But, if you happen to have been born with a particular combo of genes that predispose you to certain conditions, do you really want to test it out and see where it gets you?

*** **USEFUL FACT** *** *When stress becomes chronic, it can wreak havoc on your gut and digestive health due to decreased nutrient absorption, decreased oxygenation to your gut as much as four times less blood flow to your digestive system and decreased enzymatic output in your gut – as much as 20,000-fold! See NOTES.*

Take good care of yourself

Aim to eat, drink, sleep, and relax, all in proportion. I probably did too little of any of this, only to discover that I'm not invincible. I'm definitely catching up now. Perfecting the art of laying about has not come easy to me, but nature has its ways and I am slowly learning.

Strengthen your immune system

I never quite believed in the concept of strengthening the immune system. But after eating lotsa humble pie, I've discovered that certain therapies and actions certainly had beneficial effects and strengthened my immune system quite considerably. At some stage, the herbs rhemania, withania and rhodiola worked miracles for me. After this, removing all noises, light, and stresses wherever this was possible made a huge positive difference, even to the point where I underwent long periods of talking fasts, simply because it took more energy than I had available to think or respond to even the simplest of questions.

Get away from doomsayers

Another top priority was to take a load of my recovering organs. Also, finding a place of rest where I would no longer be a target for the labels and death sentences thrown my way by well-meaning friends in the medical industry was a huge step in the right direction.

Some of the labels included Lyme disease, Lupus, Myalgic Encephalomyelitis, chronic fatigue, Fibromyalgia, chronic pancreatitis, chronic rickettsia, ongoing and persistent Glandular Fever (Epstein-Barr virus), angina, coeliac, irritable bowel, orthostatic intolerance, chemical sensitivities, and on and on it went. And these were only some of the labels I was told to try on for size.

I am well aware that a diagnosis is needed before treatment, but I decided that all labels were an ill fit.

Sure, I was chronically fatigued and sensitive to chemicals, my pancreas was not happy, nor were my bowels. But the scary thing with labels is that once they stick, then what?

I appreciated the care and thorough investigations, but eventually all the waiting around, the cost, the prodding and poking, got me weaker and weaker with really not much of an end in sight. As I said before, at my worst I've been out of action for months and months on end; not even able to come out for a doctor's visit or test or anything at all. As soon as I got well enough for another round of investigations, the whole rigmarole would start all over again.

In the end I refused to accept any of these labels because none of them included the promise of effective treatment with an expected cure at the end. All of these labels warranted some kind of treatment to 'manage' the symptoms and illness. I resolved to do better than that and come out on the other end with a clean bill of health.

Find rest

Both the Sunshine Coast and Wide Bay Region provided me with sanctuaries where I managed to escape from the well-intentioned onslaught of medical tests and examinations, investigations and diagnosis. The upshot and outcomes of the pathology and myriad of other tests has been a merciless adding of undesirable sticky tags to my unwanted collection of medical (mis)diagnosis. Added to my woes were the tight financial restraints, which more often than not prevented me from attending necessary follow-ups.

Stay away from drugs

At some stage for instance, we discovered a wonderful alternative to antibiotic treatment with promising early positive results. However, as with all treatments, one has to follow through and continue treatment till the very end, which I was unable to do. Ordinary antibiotics have their place in medicine but they should always be used with great caution.

*** **USEFUL FACT** *** *Antibiotics kill your body's good bacteria too, which can lead to serious health risks and likely help fungi to proliferate within your body.*
In the gut live one trillion bacteria, which are known as microbiota or gut flora, and that have co-evolved in symbiosis with humans. Treatment with antibiotics can alter this symbiosis from early stages of the treatment. Although some of the changes are oscillatory and can be reversed at the end of the treatment, others seem irreversible. See NOTES.

The very basic diet I have been on for the last few years has allowed me to take a breather, and whilst perhaps not completely healing my body, at least the diet has given my family and my, by now, delicate constitution, enough rest and peace of mind to ever so gently push for further improvements.

CHAPTER TWO
WHAT MAKES ME SAY THAT THE DIET WORKS?

Many people, particularly when first diagnosed with a condition like coeliac disease, run around in desperation trying to find a diet that actually works. I know this because I've heard family and friends struggling to find the proper diet for their condition, and I've needed to create several diets over the years for various conditions for my children and myself a few times over.

Nowadays, many people seem to be suffering from all kinds of allergies, intolerances, and chemical sensitivities, more so than ever before. Cattle are more often than not fed antibiotics, and vegetable growers routinely use pesticides and artificial fertilizers. That means that our meat and vegetables as well as our environment are polluted. It's anyone's guess as to how this is affecting our bodies and gene pool. Lots of people I know are struggling like crazy in their attempts to put together a diet or menu plan that works for their particular condition.

People struggle not only because it is hard to find the right ingredients, but because whatever they are directed to buy as alternatives is so frightfully expensive.

Allergies and intolerances
are very expensive

In fact, the allergies and intolerances themselves come for free, but the diet one has to follow as a result of it is nearly always unaffordable, unless one takes out another mortgage on their house. As it stands, I don't own a house, so that wasn't an option for me. To stay alive, I simply had to find affordable alternatives, with the only other option being an early demise; I rejected that alternative.

Suitable for people with food
intolerances

A friend of ours has a granddaughter who has been diagnosed as a coeliac. Every time her granddaughter visits, our friend hits the shops to purchase gluten-free flour mixes to make cookies and pancakes and scones and so on. These mixes cost around three times what the ordinary gluten-containing mixes cost. Our friend purchases loaves of gluten-free bread for around seven bucks each. These loaves are about half the size of the loaves of bread that people without coeliac disease enjoy, with these loaves only costing around two bucks each.
I know this because I used to buy these gluten-free loaves myself.

At the moment, I cannot tolerate bread, pancakes, cookies, or scones. I cannot tolerate any of the loaves made with wheat flour, nor can I tolerate them if they are made with spelt or gluten-free flour such as corn or rice flour. What about the breads made with sprouts? Nope, I cannot tolerate them either. I cannot even tolerate the sprouts on their own. So if you were hoping that I have come up with a replacement for all these yummy things that people without health problems take for granted ... sorry, but no. I am not eating any of these sweet and scrumptious high-carb foods myself. I am simply not able to.

This diet works!

What I mean when I say that my diet works is that
a. After nearly five years on this diet, so far it seems to take care of my nutritional needs.
b. I can afford the ingredients whilst living on a limited budget.
c. I don't get hungry in between meals.
d. I don't get cravings.
e. I have pretty much maintained my weight throughout.
f. The level of intensity of many aches, pains, and cramps has diminished significantly.
g. The migraines and tummy upsets are not completely gone, but they are far less frequent.
h. There's plenty room for improvement, but I'm alive and breathing; the brain cogs are turning over once more and I'm slowly expanding my diet.

To me, that means that my diet works!

I used to have ongoing massive disabling aches and pains and cramps, which seemed to come out of nowhere and dominate my days and nights. I cannot say that I am pain free at the moment, but the pain is not all-absorbing any longer, nor is it running my life.

The same applies with the migraines, which would seemingly come out of nowhere and turn my whole body into a battlefield where light and sound and movement were bringing on the cramps and the emptying out of the spoils. Food poisoning was another regular occurrence that we have more under control now.

We discovered that my body seems to attract bugs (germs and bacteria) from a mile off and is not able to fight off infections. Over time, we came to the realisation that not only was I not able to eat what my daughters ate, but in addition, the ordinary day-to-day microbes and bacteria were trying to finish me off. As soon as my daughters divided up our kitchen utensils and so on, virtually all the food poisonings stopped. Now the girls use separate fridges, chopping boards, utensils, cutlery, crockery, pots and pans, and tea towels. With this approach, we've greatly minimised any untoward germs coming my way, and it has made a tremendous positive difference.

I still cannot tolerate any kind of grain, including rice, any kind of flour, no meat, no tofu, no tempeh, no cheese (not any kind of cheese), no eggs, no nuts, no seeds, no beans nor lentils, no potatoes, no tomatoes, no cabbage nor broccoli, and so on. So for me, as a person who has huge intolerances to the majority of foods, being able to come up with a diet that works was a major break-through.
It enabled me to stay alive.

*** **USEFUL FACT** *** *Food intolerance: The inability to fully digest a food. When your body cannot completely process a food - the result is partially digested proteins and sugars.*
This happens especially with foods like grains, milk and sugars. Protein breakdown fragments in particular cause trouble because the body does not recognise them as 'friendly'. This sets up inflammation and disrupts bodily

functions. . . causing dozens of symptoms and can develop into disease if left unattended. See NOTES.

CHAPTER THREE
WHAT IS IN THIS BOOK?

Aside from some of my history; what else am I sharing in this book? There is information about what a well-balanced diet should contain and a description on how other people have benefited from my diet. Later on, there is a discussion about various other restricted diets. After this I mention the ten ingredients I lived on for the last five years and how my diet can be easily adapted for different requirements. This is followed by a detailed outline of the various ingredients of this diet and where they can be purchased at good prices.

In truth there are 11 ingredients in my diet and the first one is prayer which I call 'oodles of faith.' I even include the Scripture verses which got me out of the emergency intake area into a medical room with prompt medical attention, and this is covered later in the book. God hears prayer; it is as simple as that.

Bonus diet

After the Afterword, I give my readers a bonus OSFA (2) diet, which tells you what I'm up to now, and it is Good News!

The diet of ten-ingredients-only that I have been on for 5 solid years I will call the low reactive OSFA (1) (One Size Fits All) diet plan. The bonus diet plan at the end of the book is what I am on now, and I call this the recovery diet OSFA (2) diet plan. This is the bonus diet. I think that the OSFA (2) diet plan is by far the better choice, but at the time I was not able to tolerate this. The only reason that I have been on a ten-ingredient-only diet is because that is all I could tolerate and not because I think it is a good idea. But it worked … for me.

The purpose of this book

Why did I write this book? I wrote this book because I know that many people suffer because of all kinds of health problems and often these problems are diet related. Obviously not always. But I wrote this book for those people who suffer from health problems due to diet related issues. My diet may be suitable for anyone who suffers from gut problems, food allergies, food intolerances and chemical sensitivities.

In addition, many conditions such as Chronic Fatigue, Fibromyalgia, Lupus, Lyme, diverticulitis and various other health problems and even menopausal symptoms are relieved when all allergens are taken out of the diet or minimised as much as possible.

I hope that my low reactive diet (OSFA 1) and bonus recovery diet (OSFA 2) will give you the inspiration, in collaboration with your health professionals, to come up with your own variation suited to your situation.

I also urge all my readers to PLEASE, PLEASE, PLEASE consider the stresses in your life and as much as possible reduce them. Because guaranteed over time, unresolved stresses will impact your health negatively.

If you think, like I did, that these stresses are unavoidable and you 'just have to suck it up,' be prepared for the eventual inevitable crumbling of your health. This is pretty much a guarantee following prolonged and unresolved stresses and tension in your life.

*** **USEFUL FACT** *** *Chronic stress can trigger symptoms and full-blown disease in your gut and contribute to conditions such as Lupus, Chronic Fatigue Syndrome, Fibromyalgia, Myalgic Encephalomyelitis and Inflammatory bowel diseases and the like. As Harvard researchers explain: "Stress (or depression or other psychological factors) can affect movement and contractions of the GI tract, cause inflammation, or make you more susceptible to infection." See NOTES.*

Easy and affordable meals

My family and I, out of necessity, researched the best of the best from the resources accessible to us today. Not only that, but because I am on a restricted budget and am not able to prepare my own meals, whatever we came up with had to be readily available, economical and easy to prepare.

At a glance, the diet may not appear to be that economical, especially because it contains organic ingredients, but when you consider that this is truly all I eat and absolutely nothing else, the diet as it is becomes quite affordable. Where I live we can source organic carrots for around $2.20 kilo pretty much all year around. I didn't start off eating organic but discovered that eating organic allowed me to introduce many more ingredients to my diet.

Some of the food gets prepared up to two days in advance and stored in the fridge for easy reheating. This means that often enough meals only need to be cooked two or three times a week. Nowadays, our soups are made in a soup maker, which takes just five minutes to prepare, and these soups are easily stored in the fridge or even frozen. We very much appreciate our Kambrook soup maker.

Easy-peasy quick meals

Some of our easiest and quickest meals are prepared when we've actually run out of fresh ingredients. This is because on those days my daughter just grabs a pack of frozen veg from the freezer, and with the help of our soup maker and a dash of miso, whips up a delicious organic soup in no time.

Invaluable information compassionate health practitioners

An invaluable list of websites and favourite people is included. One of the hardest things to come by for me in my search for health was a list of knowledgeable and compassionate health practitioners. I've created such a list, which is located at the back of this book on the thank you page. Some of the practitioners listed consult by phone, which is essential for people with delicate constitutions who may not be able to travel and are in need of specialist advice. I am humbled by and grateful for the care and dedication that my health advisers have shown me.

Both Rain-tree.com and Iherb.com deserve a special mention because the products sold by both of them are unequalled in both price and quality. In addition, they both freely provide helpful information to assist consumers determine which products to purchase.

If lentils are your thing

I've also included information on other restricted diets, starting off here with my daughter's penchant for mixing a can of tomatoes with a can of lentils, either heated as a soup or thrown together with some noodles, for breakfast, lunch and dinner, for months and months on end, seemingly with no ill effects. I would certainly never recommend this for any long-term solution. But if lentils are your thing, for a temporary solution, it doesn't really come easier or more economical than that.

CHAPTER FOUR
ABOUT OTHER RESTRICTED DIETS

LIMITED DIETS

Over the last few years, I've come across a few other diets which are rather limited, some healthy and others that are not so healthy. A healthy, balanced diet should provide us with all the carbohydrates, proteins, fat and vitamins, minerals, amino acids, and so on to give us enough fuel and building materials to support an active lifestyle. I'll list a couple of these diets to illustrate that people can get by for long periods of time with much less nutrition than we ordinarily think possible.

No fruit or veg

Vegemite diet

In 2006, the Australian Medical Journal published an article about a 22-year-old male kitchen-hand who presented with a 4-week history of extensive bruising and broken blood vessels on his legs. He had no history of any other medical conditions, except for several episodes of nosebleeds in the past few months. He was not taking any medication, and there was no known familial bleeding tendency.

On review, he had a large, tense haematoma on his left leg that was restricting his mobility, as well as a rash, which may have been present for up to 2 years. His gums were swollen and bleeding. Further examination was unremarkable.

He smoked 10–15 cigarettes daily and episodically drank large amounts of alcohol. He lived with his girlfriend. A full dietary history revealed a diet entirely comprised of Vegemite spread, cheese, bread, dry biscuits, chocolate, and a cola drink, with no fruit or vegetables whatsoever. The patient conceded that he had not tried any new foods for over 10 years, and, despite the recent diagnosis of scurvy, he was reluctant to initiate dietary change.

Humans are one of the few mammals that cannot synthesise vitamin C (ascorbic acid). Stores are readily depleted, with studies showing clinical manifestations after about a month on a vitamin C-free diet.

Because of his iron deficiency and the possibility of significant occult blood loss, he was given an immediate transfusion of packed red cells. The haemoglobin level remained stable after the transfusion. Further testing revealed a low level of vitamin C (3 μmol/L [RR, 26–85 μmol/L]), and he was prescribed oral vitamin C and iron supplements. Within a week, the condition of his legs was starting to improve. On review, 1 month later, their appearance was almost back to normal.

After ten years on a diet of Vegemite, cheese, bread, dry biscuits, chocolate and a cola drink, this young man's symptoms of scurvy cleared up within about a month. By the sound of it, it took around 8 years of living on the limited diet for these symptoms to develop.

Potatoes only

Potato Diet

Chris Voigt told Live Science that he consulted with a doctor and dietitian to confirm he could go 60 days on just potatoes. You need healthy kidneys to process the excess potassium delivered by 20 potatoes a day. You also need a store of nutrients that potatoes lack, such as vitamin A, for proper vision.

The above diet shows that one can live on a very limited diet such as potatoes only, for a certain amount of time. Voigt maintained his diet for two months, not only without ill effects, but he actually appeared to have benefited from the diet with a recorded weight loss of 21 pounds, and his cholesterol went down significantly, from 214 to 147.

Potatoes versus vegemite

The kitchen hand's diet was not quite as limited as the potato diet, but he was on his diet for ten years and his diet did not contain any fruit or vegetables. It is quite surprising that he was as healthy as he was and that he recovered as quickly as he did from the scurvy. More surprising than that was the fact that he did not seem inclined to make any dietary changes or add a multi vitamin to his diet.

Fad diets

There is a whole host of fad diets available, from cabbage soup and other low carb, to high protein, to watermelon only. Nutrition Australia had a look at some of these diets and concluded that most, if not all, of these diets seem to create problems in the long term because they are not balanced.

One of my favourite friends invites people over for dinner and reliably serves cabbage soup at her dinner parties.
That's right. JUST cabbage soup.
Yes … hmmm. I thought I may as well put this in here.
I don't know what to think about it either. Needless to say, we don't visit her much during 'cabbage season.'

I've never been one to follow fad diets, but in the past, for cleansing purposes, I've been on a carrot juice fast which contained carrots only and managed to put on 3 kilos in a period of a week and a half. What that tells me is that my metabolism was astute enough to detect 'something strange' going on, and it slowed down to the point where it completely defeated the purpose of the fast.

Another problem with an unbalanced diet is that it either keeps you hungry in between meals or craving certain foods. In the long term, we cannot count on any of these diets to provide all of the nutrients our bodies need for fuel for energy, growth, and repairs.

Mainly rice

The rice diet

If you were to be concerned about my diet not containing enough nutrients, we need to consider that people who live in Western societies generally eat too much anyway. Many of our ailments are not caused by malnutrition due to a lack of sufficient nutrients, but many in the Western world suffer from malnutrition due to overeating and over indulgence.

That's embarrassing. We literally eat ourselves sick. We spend too much money on all the wrong foods, and we follow this up with once more spending too much money and time, this time around on trying to correct the problems we created by overindulgence. It is good to keep that in mind when we devise our diet plan.

It is also good to realise that billions of people we share this planet with get by on a fairly basic rice diet, every single day of their lives. The only addition to the bowl of rice may be a little protein such as dhal or fish, tofu or tempeh. Whole nations of people live on basic rice diets, often working very long days, six or seven days a week, without falling ill or lacking basic nutrients.

*** **FUN FOOD FACT** *** *Nearly half the world's 6.6 billion population eat rice as part of their staple diet. There are more than 40,000 different varieties of rice. Rice is gluten-free and low in fat. It contains all eight essential amino acids, folic acid, and is very low in sodium and cholesterol. See NOTES.*

If I were able to tolerate rice, I could possibly devise a diet plan with only five or so ingredients in it in total, and live a perfectly healthy life, surviving on that diet.

Too much

The point I am trying to make here is that perhaps the problem is not too few ingredients, but maybe for some of us the problem is too many ingredients, leaving us with tastebuds that have been spoiled and need re-educating.

Research shows us that people who eat less tend to live longer, and being overweight is a sure recipe for suffering ailments, as well as a shorter lifespan.

Next time we open a pack of our favourite cookies, we should have a look at the ingredient list and realise that the majority of people on this planet get by with fewer ingredients than those that are listed on our pack or tin of cookies. And this is for all of their meals; breakfast, lunch and dinner combined.

Sorry to be such a spoilsport, but we don't actually need, at least for nutritional value, any of the ingredients that are listed on a pack of cookies. Without me reading any of the contents, I know that we would be better off without any of these ingredients in our system. Even when considering the 'feel-good' factor. Reality is that a glass of refreshing spring water will not only make us feel much better than any cookie ever will, but in the long run, it will also benefit us more.

Biblical fast

Forty-day fast

I was raised a Catholic and when I grew up, the emphasis was more on church attendance than on reading the Bible. Once I opened my Bible and started reading it; I couldn't stop. Among many other things I discovered a few interesting facts about fasting.

The Bible lists a number of cases where people have fasted for forty days without any ill effects reported. These fasts appeared to have been purification, or what we call cleansing fasts today. The first occasion listed in the Bible is where Moses fasted before he went up Mount Sinai to receive the Commandments. The second fast mentioned is where Elijah the prophet fasted straight after the drought. Jesus also fasted for forty days in the desert before he began his ministry.

Check with your health practitioner

Nowadays, we're always told to check with our health practitioner before we commence any kind of health program or fast, and I think that is an excellent idea. Don't just do what I did. Nor should you blindly follow anyone else, either. Experiment, carefully, and take this book as a warning not to take your health for granted. My wish for my readers is that my diet may give you the inspiration to find out what works for you. Talk with your health provider and plan a diet and health routine tailored exactly to *your* needs.

Certain diets work for certain people for a particular period of time. Some people get better on a high protein diet and others get better on a low protein diet. It all depends on your condition, environment, genes and what stage of your life you're in.

Food for thought

Added bonus

I don't do my own cooking, but with this diet, the meal preparation literally takes as long as it takes to cook a carrot.

I don't do my own shopping either, but if I did, it would be so easy on my diet, with all the ingredients set for the week. For anyone on a fixed and limited budget that indeed is a blessing.

Limited as my diet may seem, another definite perk is that for the last few years, whenever I've tried to add new ingredients, I quickly find out if I can manage the new addition to my diet or not.

Prior to being on this diet, I was struggling to find out if it was the yoghurt that mucked me up, or the bread, or eating both of them at the same meal, or what? Because the diet I am on works for me, I can tell very quickly if the new food is a winner or a no-go.

Another added bonus from following my special diet has come as a bit of surprise to me. What I've noticed over time is that my tears have dried up. There has been plenty to cry about with the sheer physical pain and decline that I experienced, compounded by financial ruin and the accompanying predictable crumbling of close relationships.

The stresses in my life helped to kick in menopause around ten years early. Well, let's say ten years earlier than my Mum's or my sister's. It wasn't till I went on my ten-ingredient-only diet that the mood swings, which can be brought on by the hormonal changes, evened out and some sense of calm and peace returned to my life.

I experienced much grief when I contemplated the loss of my life as I knew it, which included the dissipating of my career and my standing in society. The list goes on. But with my diet, there are no tears. I have tackled an abundance of challenges followed by miraculous recoveries and on this diet, not even a sniffle.

Teary eyed

In the past, I found that even the tiniest amount of chocolate, such as, for instance, a quarter of a little piece of white (my favourite) or pure chocolate or a sliver of dried pineapple would bring on the tears and relentless despondency. A few grains of sugar ingested in any form used to reliably open the floodgates. Food for thought, I think. I know many people, and my Mum was one of them, who love chocolate and can enjoy slabs of it in blissful euphoria without suffering any kind of ill effects.

I am simply not one of those people. I cannot have chocolate or any amount of sugar in any form without descending into an emotional abyss of anguish followed by streams of tears. Not so for my Mum or Dad, nor my siblings. All of them enjoyed, and as far as I know still enjoy, sweets such as cakes and cookies and tarts with cream and chocolate galore.

CHAPTER FIVE
WHAT DOES THE DIETITIANS ASSOCIATION SAY ABOUT THE OSFA DIET PLAN?

CHOOSE A VARIETY OF FOODS

The Dietitians Association of Australia tells us to choose a variety of foods including breads, cereals, fruits and vegetables, moderate amounts of low-fat dairy foods, and lean meats or alternatives; and small amounts of poly-unsaturated or mono-unsaturated fats and oils.

The Dietitians Association tells us to aim for at least twenty food items or ingredients daily. The Association tells us that it has been shown that food variety has a direct correlation with nutritional value. As bonus advice, the Dietitians Association throws in the recommendation for people to be physically active, and to do so in a way that is enjoyable.

Sound advice, I would say, and alongside increasing my diet with a wider variety of foods, I am also working on the physically active part. I've pretty much perfected the art of laying about, and it may just be time to move on to the next phase of my recovery. My mind and spirit are ready, and time will tell if the rest of me is ready to play ball.

Over the past few years, we've run my diet past three dietitians, and only the last one made some recommendations for added nutrition. The upshot of the suggestion was to add a multi mineral and vitamin tablet a day to make sure that I receive all of the necessary nutrition. My vitamin B intake and some of the minerals appeared low. This is no surprise, given that I only managed to eat and digest small amounts of anything at any time.

A range of stuff showed up in my last mineral test, and I intend to tackle this by removing, wherever possible, all stressors from my life and supplement as suggested by Dr Wilson and Dr Lizon (See NOTES). As part of a health care plan it is not a bad idea to, every now and then, do a mineral test, and this way stay on top of health issues before they get out of control.

One dietitian suggested that I curtail my yoghurt intake. I followed up on this advice. Acidophilus capsules don't agree with me, however, nor have the supplements I've taken so far. Yoghurt can be replaced with quark or buttermilk, homemade or store-bought soy yoghurt, and kefir. I am currently looking into that.

Up till my hospital stay I had been eating what everyone would consider a healthy diet. We used to get our vegetables from the Farmers Market in Noosa. Organic vegetables at this market were, at the time, better priced than the ordinary produce at our local super market. Every weekend we used to buy baskets overflowing with fresh produce, gluten-free bread, and organic eggs. And yet, due to my genetic predisposition and the years of antibiotics (ab)use, all it took was a house move, for my delicate constitution to crumble in one big heap.

CHAPTER SIX
IS THE ONE SIZE FITS ALL OSFA DIET PLAN A MAGIC BULLET?

CURE FOR ALL?

Is my diet a magic bullet? Most certainly not, and I would hate to think that anyone else would be on this diet for five years like I have been. At the same time, however, this diet has really served me very well and continues to do so today. Knowing that there are so many people out in the world with dietary challenges, it feels selfish to keep my diet to myself.

The other day I was reading a post on an internet forum where young university students were discussing what life was like after having been diagnosed as a coeliac. Many found that the sugars in milk and apples caused them problems as well. These young students were really struggling with their health on a limited budget, with limited knowledge and limited time, trying to make it all work. Many universities provide excellent information on how to prepare nutritious and affordable meals, but few, if any, of these booklets take into consideration the many food intolerances that are suffered by students nowadays.

I have no qualifications as a medical person, dietitian, or a naturopath. I have just managed to stay alive after I had in succession, heart failures, severe pancreatic attacks, an inoperable ruptured appendix and septicaemia, together with intolerance to many foods and antibiotics. When I returned home from the hospital, I was not able to keep any food or liquid down, and for various reasons, partially to do with the collapse of my carefully stacked credit card empire and inability to get up from bed, there was only limited medical help available; provided mainly through phone consultations.

It was only hours after the removals truck had left that an ambulance raced me to the local hospital emergency department. The fact that we were brand new in town with doctors reluctant to add a patient seemingly 'knocking on heaven's door' to their books probably had something to do with my daughters' inability to secure a doctor's home visit for me.

What did we learn from this experience? Prayer works. It works real well for my children and I. The love and care of my kids went a long way too. The homeopathic care I received was truly invaluable. Hugs for the couple of doctors who made themselves and their medical advice available to us over the phone.

Is my diet a cure for all? I doubt it very much. I do believe, however, that many people who are struggling with their diet may be inspired by the possibilities I present here in this book. And it is my hope and prayer that together with their health provider, people will be able to come up with alternatives instead of struggling on a daily basis with their diet.

Ecstatically happy

So I'm still not up and running like I used to, and frankly, I don't intend to ever get back to the mad rush that used to be my life, with 24/7 duties and no rest, peace, or joy factored in. I am content though. To tell you the truth, I'm ecstatically happy that I'm still around, and I thank my Creator every single day for keeping an eye on me and mine.

Acne problems

To get back to the diet. Thus far, I have shared my diet with two other people. One had acne problems, which cleared up within one month on the diet. The young adolescent assured me that if she were to stay on the diet and simply expand it with a larger variety of vegetables and protein, her face would be without blemish. This young woman appears to have sugar intolerance, and the lure of chocolate and sugary foods occasionally gets the better of her, which results in the odd pimple here and there. The severe acne problems she suffered in the past are now, seemingly, gone for good.

She, like the university students I encountered on an internet forum, also cannot tolerate any apple or fig in the diet, and instead she get her vitamin C from a multivitamin, which includes iron. She cannot tolerate yoghurt and instead has rice puffs (the sugarless kind with an ingredients list that read 100% puffed rice) with milk. She also prefers tofu, tempeh, and egg instead of the fish I eat.

Depression

The other young girl I shared my diet with experienced quite severe mood swings. However, as soon as she has been on my diet for a few days, her moods settled and become more stable. The longer she is on the diet, the better she is able to handle the ups and down that come her way.

This young lady has a penchant for carbs, any kind of carbs and when not on the diet, she'll scoff down a big (serving) bowl of rice, just plain rice, followed by a big bowl of noodles, just plain noodles, just for the carbs hit. It is nothing to her to devour one whole loaf of bread on her own in a matter of hours. Just plain bread, no toppings nor butter. It is really a sight to behold. When on the diet, Candidate Two prefers tofu, cottage cheese, and lentils instead of the fish I eat.

I mention the two examples given above as an illustration to show how easily adaptable the diet I eat is, by simply swapping the protein for another kind of protein and adding in other sorts of vegetables and/or grains/beans or lentils if required or desired.

It is very likely that the acne and depression accompanied by a partiality for carb hits are caused by underlying health problems. Problems that need to be addressed by a medically qualified doctor or health professional. Meanwhile, until these problems are addressed in some way, the diet works quite well as an interim measure.

Diet plan?

Maybe diet plan is too big a word for the few ingredients I manage to stay alive on. How did it come about? 100% trial and error.

After I returned from hospital, I literally could not keep down water. Slowly, very slowly, with trial and error, soups and purees, countless food poisonings (due to my delicate and frail gut), eventually we settled on the following diet plan, which we'll call the One Size Fits All or OSFA (1) DIET.

CHAPTER SEVEN
OSFA (1) DIET

Breakfast – lunch – dinner

- ½ cooked carrot
- ¼ cooked sweet potato
- ½ cup cooked green beans
- ½ spoon of coconut oil and a little salt
- 2 spoons filled with kosher fish

- ½ cup plain yoghurt
- ¼ apple and dried ½ fig

- 2 digestives (one dairy) with each meal

Drinks

Drink in between meals only, one hour before or after meals.

- Herbal teas; horsetail, nettle, dandelion, sage, spearmint, sleepy tea
- Filtered water with a spoonful of Himalayan rock salt brine
- Filtered water with ½ spoonful of barley- or wheat-grass or alfalfa powder

Lunch variation

When tolerated, the cooked vegetables can be substituted for lunch with:

- 7 raw snow peas
- A handful of snow pea sprouts

- . 5 slices of cucumber
- . Petals, avocado, pawpaw when in season

The above food is all I've eaten (tolerated) since early 2009. Nothing else. As in really, nothing else whatsoever.

How did I come to this diet?

This low reactive diet plan came about after months of prayer and trial and error and we came to this bit-by-bit. As I explained earlier, when I came out of the hospital I tolerated nothing, not even water. Whenever we tried to get me back onto my previous 'healthy diet' of fresh raw greens my whole system would cramp up and was unable to digest any of it.

Once we realised that I wasn't able to digest most of the foods I was used to, we looked up what babies eat and found that, for instance, mashed banana was too sweet but mashed carrot worked. Thoroughly boiled sweet potato, the orange kind was good too, as were green beans. I wasn't able to digest anything raw. And I wasn't able to tolerate any dairy.

First off, I started with;

1. Carrot
2. Sweet potato
3. Green beans
4. Kosher fish

The kosher fish was just a couple of teaspoons per meal. Keep in mind that I was just lying in bed. And anyone who would like to try a diet similar to this whilst working, would need to increase the quantities.

Eventually someone mentioned 'digestives' to us. We found 'digestives' which help with the digestion of dairy foods as well as other foods. As soon as I introduced one dairy digestive into the mix I was able to eat a small amount of unsweetened yoghurt. This helped with the gut flora which needed to be re-established after I'd been on antibiotics for a long time.

*** **USEFUL FACT** *** *Digestive enzymes are substances produced by our bodies that help us to digest the foods we eat. These enzymes are secreted by the various parts of our digestive system and they help to break down food components such as proteins, carbohydrates, and fats. As we age and due to illness, the ability to produce these enzymes decreases and we may have to supplement our diet with enzymes to be able to properly absorb our food. See NOTES.*

I mention that my diet was dairy free and indeed for quite a while it was, till we discovered the dairy digestives. However if dairy does not work for you, as it did not for me either for a while; yoghurt nowadays can be purchased as soy yoghurt, coconut or lactose free yoghurt.

5. Yoghurt

The other digestive (both are mentioned under notes at the back of this book) helped me digest the tiny bits of apple and fig, which we eventually introduced after at least a couple of years on the above diet. We started off with just a sliver of apple and a quarter of a fig and slowly over time increased these amounts to half an apple and a whole fig at meal times.

6. Apple
7. Fig

I probably lived on those first seven ingredients, as described above, for a period of two or three years. Most of the time I had the three vegetables in a soup (or steamed), with the fish on the side and, once the yoghurt and fruit was introduced, I had the yoghurt, apple and fig as desert; for breakfast, lunch and dinner.

Oh the joy!

I cannot even begin to describe the joy that we all experienced when we had the meals 'sorted' without gut problems and dramas. It took an enormous amount of stress out of our daily life to be able to purchase food in advance and know that I finally got the minimum of nutrition so that I would at least not go backwards.

This diet plan I was on, stopped the cramps, stopped the indigestion, stopped the migraines, the rashes and it stopped all sorts of health problems that I was experiencing. Finally I could eat in peace, without fear.

Eventually with the help of the digestives I was able to digest snow peas and sprouts, and cucumber also. We started off with tiny bits at a time. Like really, half a snow pea and then not at all for two or three days and then again half a snow pea and nothing for a couple of days and then one whole snow pea … yeah victory and so on.

8. Raw snow peas
9. Snow pea sprouts
10. Cucumber

I know this sounds pretty crazy, but this truly was my reality. If I didn't follow this system I would reliably end up with either massive cramping, migraines, vomiting, diarrhea or a combination of all of these.

Some people would indicate to me that it was all in my head. I just wish that someone would have been able to convince my body of that.

The above shows that I wasn't on all ten ingredients for 5 years but that they were slowly introduced one at a time. Initially, after I ruptured my appendix, first weeks and then months went by where we were at a complete loss as to what to do because at first my body literally would vomit up water and not tolerate it.

As I am writing this down, it seems pretty extreme to me and nearly unbelievable, but this truly is what happened. My daughters phoned around for a home visit both before as well as after my hospital stay. I am not surprised that doctors would not come out for a home visit but instead told my daughters to call for an ambulance. As it was, after my hospital stay, the ambulance ride would probably have been enough to finish me off.

What's next?

I'm now working up to adding in a multivitamin, minerals, and extra amino acids. On occasion, I take garlic tea. With the meals, we add in a few bits of onion, a little quinoa, Irish moss, and so on. I love coreopsis, which are gorgeous-looking yellow flowers, in the same family as buttercups and daisies, which to me look like little sun rays, but I don't always tolerate them.

So there you have it. My special diet, without sweets other than a little fig and certain types of apple, works for me. I know that there are people, as I used to be, who would not be able to tolerate the apple or the fig or the carrot, due to the relatively high sugar content. In the past, I couldn't tolerate it either without candida rearing its ugly head with accompanying migraines and all sorts of trouble. If you find that you are not able to tolerate these food items, it should not be too hard to replace these food items with ones that are tolerable.

For instance, during pumpkin season we now replace the sweet potato with butternut pumpkin and Jarrahdale pumpkin. We also exchange the orange carrots for purple ones and yellow ones whenever they are available.

I've also left out the oil and don't have any oil of any kind at the moment. I discovered that because of my pancreatic problems no oil means no pain in that area. Another improvement!

Guidance through prayer

It is true, when I said earlier that the diet came about 100% by trial and error. What is also true is that I received a lot of guidance with prayer. The problem was that I hadn't exercised my knees much, and even though I received wonderful responses to my prayers, my follow-up left a lot to be desired.

For instance, one night I went to sleep asking for a solution to the infections that seemed to plague me non-stop. I woke up in the middle of the night thinking, 'God says E, 6 times 3.' Nice little rhyme, easy to remember, and a little intriguing. Naturally, I didn't recall it in the morning and it was not till weeks later that this prompting popped back into my mind.

At breakfast one day we were discussing dreams and prayers. Propped up against my pillows whilst chewing my bit of apple, I suddenly remembered the intense prayer for a solution to the infections, and just as I was about to open my mouth to say that I was still waiting for an answer, I remembered the little rhyme. Call me cotton brain if you like, but this happened a lot to me. I would intensely pray for a solution and completely miss the answer for weeks, if not months, on end.

I was not only dopey, but also untrained and unfamiliar with prayers being answered so readily and easily. I would often get an answer and not act upon it for quite a while.

Once I remembered the little rhyme I said it out loud, "God Says E, 6 times 3." What does that mean girls? I looked around, and next to me on my bedside table was an orange little bottle of Goldenseal extract. Ha! (G)olden(S)eal (E)xtract. Tada!

Now you probably wonder why this was such a revelation, because obviously, if this bottle was on my bedside table I was already taking this supplement? Well, no. I tried, but hadn't been able to take it because every time I took a dose I would end up with a massive migraine.

Goldenseal extract is sometimes prescribed to help with the germ E coli, which of course had come into play with the septicaemia. It may have been mentioned to me by the friendly homeopath, I cannot remember, and we may have ordered it from Iherb. But the thing was that this supplement had been of no use to me because I was not able to tolerate it … till the answer to my prayer.

Once I remembered the little rhyme of 'God Says E, 6 times 3,' I decided to ignore the dosage instructions on the bottle, which was way more than I could tolerate, and took 3 drops at a time, 6 times a day. It did not take very long after this for me to be able to sit up more in bed without feeling nauseous and dizzy. Till that stage I had mainly been lying in bed not doing much of anything in particular because sitting up had been too much of an effort to me.

*** USEFUL FACT *** *Goldenseal's ability as a "natural antibiotic" has given this herb a great reputation in the herbal lore. Digestive secretions in the stomach are increased by taking the remedies made from the goldenseal. The remedy also has an astringent action on the mucous membranes lining the gut; this checks the spread of inflammation in the area at the same time. Do not use for prolonged period of time. See NOTES.*

And so little by little, step by step, I recovered eetsy weenie tiny bits at a time. This particular answer to a prayer taught me to ignore the dosages given on bottles because they were always too large for me. I learned to take things one drop at a time, even to the point where I would put one drop on my wrist and wait for a couple of days to see if there was a reaction, and after this maybe have a drop in a glass of water and wait to see if there was a reaction, and so on.

I had already learned that extracts were the way to go for me because they get absorbed easier and can be purchased without any additives. But many of these extracts were simply too potent for me to handle ... till I learned to take it really easy. Literally one drop at a time.

It was in the same way that the trial and error with the diet came about. Trying out one bite at a time. Literally take one bite of carrot and wait for a day or so to see if there was a negative reaction. I know this sounds crazy, and indeed my life was pretty crazy. Crazy good, I am still breathing! And I am still around!

Preparation

As said before, the vegetables can be baked, boiled, mashed, juiced, or served raw. People with a delicate digestive system are probably better off having the vegetables steamed or boiled.

My vegetables are cut into similar-size chunks and placed in an enamel-coated cast iron cooking pot boiled with around half a cup of water, as well as a tablespoon of Himalayan salt brine.
The whole preparation takes around ten to fifteen minutes. Once in a while, some fresh or dried basil or coriander herb is added. By the time the vegetables are cooked, all the water has disappeared.

Whilst the vegetables are cooking, yoghurt gets placed in a small bowl and garnished with slivers of apple and fig slices. A couple of spoonfuls of fish are placed in another small bowl, by which time the vegetables are cooked and served with ½ a spoonful of cold-pressed virgin coconut oil.

This meal has taken care of all my nutritional needs for five years.

Note: In 2014, we invested in a $70 soup maker. It now takes five minutes to chop up the veg and after 20 minutes, the soup maker delivers and keeps warm for us a yummy soup, blended, or whatever else we fancy. There is no need for any stirring or to keep an eye on it. What is also nice about the soup maker is that, because the device is airtight, none of the nutrients escape through the lid and go wafting through your kitchen. This means that all the goodies stay in the soup where they belong.

Intolerances

Initially, I wasn't able to tolerate snow peas, paw-paw, or avocado, but by trying minute quantities, little by little, eventually I was able to incorporate some at lunchtime.
To begin with, after my hospital stay, I also could not tolerate the yoghurt, but then we discovered the dairy digestives, and when I take them, I can have half a cup of yoghurt at a time. Anything more than that and my system gets overloaded. Probiotics would be a good idea, but once more, no go.

Initially I couldn't tolerate the apple or fig either; I reckon I must have been sweet enough. But eventually, starting with minute amounts, I could tolerate a little every now and then. At present, I am fine with the amounts described above.

It appears that the years of antibiotic medications, and in particular the medical trial, which prescribed me cocktails of antibiotics, well and truly mucked up a few things in my system, including the delicate balance of gut flora. Getting my gut back to normal has been a bit of a challenge.

The severe pancreatic attack I suffered all those years ago came about because one day I took antibiotics at the same time as probiotics. My pancreas, by then quite delicate, after enduring multiple antibiotic cocktails for months on end, protested loudly and said, "I'm outta here." It nearly finished me off, but not quite. So I'm back fighting, but naturally, I'm very cautious these days with probiotics for that reason.

Nutritional analysis

I won't go through the nutritional analysis of all the foods contained on the OSFA (1) DIET because as I said before, it works for me. But just for the heck of it, if we look at the nutritional analysis of only the sweet potato, we find that this is near enough a super food.

Sweet potato has one of the greatest sources of beta-carotene of all vegetables, and a cup of cooked sweet potato contains over 300% of our daily-required vitamin A. Sweet potato has plenty vitamin C, potassium, calcium, and carbohydrates, and is a good source of fibre too. Sweet potato is also a rare low-fat source of vitamin E and contains a good mix of vitamins, including B1, B2, B3, B5, B6, and even K, a wide range of amino acids, as well as minerals including folate, iron, magnesium and manganese, and all that with a relatively low glycemic index of only 17.

Adjusting the diet for specific needs.

Vegan and/or dairy Intolerant

Adjusting the diet for a vegan could be easily arranged by replacing the kosher fish with lentils, tofu, or tempeh and the yoghurt with soy or coconut yoghurt, almond, rice, or soy milk.

Vegetarian

Adjusting the diet for vegetarian needs could be done by replacing the kosher fish with eggs, cheese, or beans.

For fructose mal-absorption, anti-candida

The apple and fig can be replaced with other fruits that contain lower levels of sugar, such as berries, rock melon, pawpaw, apricots or plums, and a sprinkling of nuts.

Meat eaters

Meat eaters can enjoy the fish, or replace the kosher fish with any kind of meat, turkey, or chicken.

Super sensitive people

If you're anything like me, you purchase and consume organic whenever possible. And it may be worth looking into supplementing your diet for as long as you need with pre-digested lactose-free baby formula powders (ask your chemist). I've only recently started to supplement with this and found that the corn syrup did not agree with me, but I am looking forward to trying one without it.

Elimination diet

If anyone is following a restricted diet with the intent to figure out which foods cause adverse reactions, the trick is to start off with few ingredients and slowly add in one ingredient at a time, whilst monitoring the effects. A good rule of thumb is to only introduce a new ingredient every three to four days.

All diet variations

All diet variations can be played around with by minimising or increasing portion sizes, adding in and rotating vegetable kinds, boiling, baking, roasting, or steaming them, and varying the kind of fruits, proteins, and oils. Various grains, breads, rice, and pasta can be added into the mix if there is an increased energy requirement and they are tolerated. Multiple herbs and spices can be used for added flavour.

All people on whatever diet variation, as mentioned previously, would benefit if they were to add a daily multivitamin and mineral to their diet.

As much as naturopaths and dietitians may like us to be able to obtain all nutrients from our diet, the ugly truth is that much of the soils we grow our foods in are depleted and many of our waters polluted. We use a myriad of chemicals nowadays, which can interfere with nutrient absorption. And some of us have underlying medical conditions and/or certain genetic predispositions, which can prevent our body from utilising and assimilating certain vitamins or minerals. Over time, this can affect our health negatively. A little extra help in the form of a basic multivitamin and mineral may not be a bad idea.

Moo .. consider this seriously

Ordinary grasses from the paddock contain all of the nutrition that are needed for health and growth. How do I know that? Think rhinoceros, think horse, think cow. Over the last 6 months, I've had the privilege to see a 20 kg foal grow into a healthy 150 kilo pony by thriving solely on her mother's milk and grass. This is apart from the occasional mouth full of dirt, plastic, leaves and twigs and the intermittent guzzle of water. I'm not the only one who is big on grass; read Ann Wigmore's story for the full low down on the nutritional value of flowers, wheatgrass, and other grasses.

Sure, human beings aren't like cows, horses, or rhinoceroses. To gain perspective on the various diets and foods available, however, all we have to realise is that a meat eater eats the cow, a vegetarian drinks the milk, and a vegan munches the grass. Ultimately, all the nutrients came from the grass. It's simply a matter of preference and how processed you like your food.

*** **USEFUL FACT** *** *Wheatgrass is a good source of Protein and Potassium, and a very good source of Dietary Fibre, Vitamin A, Vitamin C, Vitamin E (Alpha Tocopherol), Vitamin K, Thiamin, Riboflavin, Niacin, Vitamin B6, Pantothenic Acid, Iron, Zinc, Copper, Manganese and Selenium. See NOTES.*

Digestive enzymes

Digestive enzymes are another useful dietary aid for those among us on any type of diet who cannot always easily digest all foods. Our family eats kosher and we purchase vegan and vegetarian digestive enzymes. We buy vegan or vegetarian enzymes because many of the readily available digestive enzymes contain porcine pancreatin, which has been derived from pig.

Enzymes can be purchased to help digest any kind of food, such as, for instance, fatty and oily substances, or those containing gluten, or cruciferous foods, or dairy, or lectins, and more.

CHAPTER EIGHT
I STAYED ALIVE!

IT COULD HAVE GONE WRONG

When the ambulance came to our house, I was in so much pain that I was not able to walk and pretty much had to slip my way down the staircase with my bum, one step at a time. I think at the bottom of the stairs the guys got me on a stretcher, but I cannot really remember. When we got to the hospital, the ambulance officers were told to wait with me on the stretcher at the emergency check-in area, which was chockers on a weekend night. In fact, as we found out later, it had been one of the most horrendous nights at the local hospital, with casualties and deceased being brought in from a car crash only a little while after I checked in on the night of July 18 in the year 2008.

It could have gone wrong when I experienced hideous pain and my girls phoned around but weren't able to secure a doctor's home visit for me.

But what happened instead was that between their frantic phone calls, a friend of the family phoned to check in with us and asked how the house move was going. Did we arrive safely and all that? My daughters told Michael about their mum near enough passing out from the pain in her gut, and he implored them to phone an ambulance. Michael was a friend we had met through my brother, and Michael prayed for us. Chances are that if Michael had not phoned, prayed for us, and encouraged my girls to get an ambulance, it could have gone wrong. But it didn't and I stayed alive. Angels truly exist and one of them made a lifesaving call on July 18 in the year 2008. Don't tell me that angels don't exist.

As I said, it was one of the most horrendous nights in the history of our local hospital, the nurses kept telling me that this was one of, if not their worst, 'full moon nights.' As a result of this being an extremely busy night at the hospital, I was not paid much attention and placed on the stretcher right next to the glistening, noisily-vibrating fridges filled with drinks. The noise was more than I could handle and the girls asked if I could please be moved elsewhere. This was refused by the ambulance officers.

Both the pain and the noise, as well as the light, were unbearable to me, and my eldest daughter continued to make attempts to have me moved to a more quiet location. Her attempts were noted in the report as her being obnoxious and uncooperative. The kid was trying to save her mum's life, for crying out loud!

Oh sing unto the Lord

As I could feel my life ebbing away, I'm not sure who started it, but all of a sudden the three of us were singing the Scripture Songs which I had created a few months prior to help us with our house move. It went something like this,

Oh Sing unto the Lord a new song,
O sing unto the Lord a new song,
O sing unto the Lord
All the earth

It came even to pass when the singers were as one
To make one sound to be heard on praising
And thanking the Lord
And when they lifted up their voice
The glory of the Lord had filled the house

Praise the Lord all ye nations
Praise him all ye people
For his merciful kindness is great toward us;
And the truth of the Lord
Endureth forever
Oh praise ye the Lord
Praise Yah

By the word of the Lord were the heavens made
And all the host of them
By the breath of his mouth
Let all the earth fear the Lord
And all the inhabitants be in awe

For he spake and it was done
He commanded and it stood fast
Please forsake not the work of thine own hands
God's word shall not return void

We waited patiently for the Lord
He lifted us out of the miry clay
And set our feet upon a rock
And established our goings

Many shall see and trust in the Lord
Many shall see and trust in the Lord
Oh many shall see and trust in the Lord
Amen

We walk with God like Enoch did
And we wanna be no more like Enoch did
For God took him and we wanna be like him
But thy will be done

In earth as in heaven
In earth as in heaven
In earth as in heaven
Thy will be done.

I really cannot remember if we got as far as this or if we sang even more than this. But what I can remember is that in no time at all, after we started singing, I was wheeled out of the emergency admission room into a nearby emergency treatment private room. This is where we spent most the night, and I was closely monitored by machines and doctors as the diseased and casualties of an accident were brought in and treated all around me. This happened with accompanying screams of a teenage girl begging the surgeons 'to please not cut off her legs.'

It could have gone wrong but it didn't

Blood was taken, scans made, and tests performed, and this is also where the doctors told my daughters that it was too risky to operate on me. So once more it could have gone wrong, but it didn't and I stayed alive!

Eventually, as the first light peeked into the hospital windows, I was wheeled into another private room for hourly monitoring and investigations began in earnest. Many more times it could have gone wrong, but it didn't. For instance, when the nurses were about to inject dye into my veins for the scans, and we only just prevented potentially toxic material being injected into my extremely sensitive and over-reactive veins.

The scans showed that my appendix had gone into hiding and all that could be seen were adhesions. Adhesions are like a type of scar tissue, or rather bands of fibrous tissue that can form between abdominal tissues and organs as a result of trauma such as surgery, infection, and for instance, a ruptured appendix. Abdominal adhesions can cause tissues and organs in the abdominal cavity to stick together.

Before I came to hospital I had experienced many adverse reactions to antibiotics and my body vehemently protested against the antibiotics, which were administered to me through a drip. Everything got continuously expelled from both ends. As soon as it came in, it went out. It could have gone wrong, but it didn't and I stayed alive.

*** **USEFUL FACT** *** *Side effects, allergies and reactions to antibiotics are not that unusual. Common side effects are rashes, diarrhea, abdominal pain,* *nausea/vomiting, hypersensitivity, dizziness. See NOTES.*

After one sleepless night in the hospital, my eldest daughter phoned around during the next night to find appropriate help for me, because she could see that the treatment I received was not necessarily doing me a lot of good. This drew the attention of some other doctors, and I ended up with a team around my bed discussing what would be the best way to go.

For a little while morphine became my best friend, but just the same it took days for my tummy to stop resembling a plank, and the relentless heaving and nonstop emptying of my bowels was taking its toll. I had to get outta here.

My girls prayed and I prayed. I had asked for the drip to be taken out, and it was agreed that the drip would be taken out to see how I would cope, and if it were possible for me to go home to recover further so that eventually I could be operated on and my appendix removed.

Raise me up please

I was desperate to get out of the hospital and back home and prayed with all my might. In some church leaflet a little while ago I had read about the Lord lifting people up and raising them higher. To be truthful, I didn't quite know what that meant, but I liked the sound of it, so I went, "Father, if you could raise me up and lift me higher and higher, please. High enough to get out of here and back home with my girls. Not beyond the clouds as yet, but high enough to get out of here, please."

I quite liked the way that sounded and repeated this a few times, and then fell asleep. The next morning my drip was taken out, and, relishing my new-found freedom, I was waving my arms up and down beside the bed when I abruptly knocked some knob. Curiosity got the better of me, and as I pressed the knob, the bed started to move up. I giggled and pressed again. Up it went. And again and again, in no time my bed was up so high that my hands touched the ceiling. My giggles became an unstoppable laugh. Mary, the cleaning lady, came in without me noticing. All of a sudden I realised that she was cleaning beneath the bed. When she was finished she looked up at me and said, 'You can come down again.'

I giggled a bit more and asked her, "Did you know that these beds go up so high?" She smiled at me and said, "Yep, we use it all the time. Although most of the new beds don't go up as high as yours; you have one of the last of the older models." And out she went to continue her round of cleaning.

Within a minute I was back touching the ceiling, and I was still there when my medical team came in a little while later. The Registrar, surrounded by nurses and a couple of other doctors, looked up and asked, "How are you feeling today?"

I grinned back at him, "On top of the world, high as a kite, I've never been better."

I was back home the next day.

CHAPTER NINE
WHERE TO PURCHASE?

Once I got back home, the girls eventually managed to secure a visit from the homeopath and the rest is history.

A family member gave helpful advice over the phone, which eventually helped to sort out some of the bowel problems. This was as simple as eating grated apple which had been sitting around for long enough to get a little brown. An old wives' tale has it that the pectin oxidizes and you're getting the same ingredient found in many over-the-counter diarrhoea medicines. I don't know if this is true, but it sure did the trick for me.

It took months and months before we settled on a diet which seemed to work for me. I lost a fair bit of weight, and at times it was touch and go. Once we managed to keep the infections under control and once I stopped having food poisonings, I started to make progress and little by little started to get better.

The ingredients necessary for my low reactive OSFA (1) diet are easily accessible to anyone.

Where do we obtain the ingredients for my meals?

I haven't actually been out shopping for a long time now, but all of the ingredients for breakfast, lunch, and dinner are purchased from our local grocery store. When available and affordable, we buy organic.

Our local grocery store sells a lovely Sleepy Time vanilla tea that is from Celestial Seasonings. The online store IHERB sells a whole range of the Celestial Seasoning products, including a Sleepy Time Extra. Both these teas are kosher.

The horsetail, nettle, dandelion, sage, and spearmint tea we purchase from IHERB at between ten and fifteen dollars for half a kilo from either STARWEST or FRONTIER herbs. The same goes for the barley, wheatgrass, and alfalfa powders.

We always buy everything local, unless the price difference is so great that it becomes lunacy to do 'the right thing.' If the choice is to pay nearly 5 dollars for 29 gram/20 teabags of non-organic tea as opposed to $10 for half a kilo of organic tea, I can only go with what makes sense and order the organic tea to be sent all the way across the globe for a fraction of what my local store charges me.

The digestive enzymes I use are NOW FOODS Dairy Digest Complete and NOW FOODS Optimal Digestive Complete. The recommended dose is two of each at mealtime. But either because I eat small meals or because I combine them both, I only seem to need one of each during mealtime. That means that a jar of 30 capsules lasts me for one whole month. Both are ordered from IHERB.

You drink salty water?

Yes, I drink salty water, and with good reason.

Some seventeen years ago, I found myself hooked up to intravenous fluids in a hospital room because I had fainted due to dehydration and sunstroke after a heatwave kind of day in an amusement park on the Gold Coast. The hastily-phoned ambulance added the bells and whistles to our otherwise fun-filled family outing.

The dehydration was severe enough that after an hour or so of unfruitful poking around my shrivelled-up veins by hospital nurses, I was transferred to a private hospital where a drip was inserted under local anaesthetic. The saline going in too fast seemed to have caused the resulting double pneumonia, but that is a different story for another day. This event was part of a kaleidoscope of events triggering my subsequent decline in health.

The second time I found myself hooked up to a drip was around five years ago, after I'd been admitted to The Bay's Hospital Emergency Department. Ominous signs in the hospital grounds prohibiting children playing in the garden because of venomous reptiles added to our sense of foreboding at the time of my admission. Our apprehension proved to be correct when I was diagnosed with septicaemia and a ruptured appendix.

What I learned from these episodes on a drip is that my skin loves all that extra moisture, in the form of saline, percolating through my veins. Saline is another word for salty water. On average, our body consists of two thirds water; even more for babies and children. This extra fluid explains, at least in part, those appealing, glowing, chubby, red, early childhood cheeks.

Researcher and doctor David Bell did a trial on twenty-five of his patients and found that some of the severely disabled ones, such as those who were confined to bed, were able to return to work after having been put on a saline drip. I would consider this option if it weren't for the infection rate, which excludes people who are intolerant to antibiotics from this kind of therapy.

Keeping myself well hydrated with filtered water infused with Himalayan rock salt brine is as close as I can get to sample a smidgen of the benefits of the therapy prescribed by Dr David Bell.

I have also discovered that with the right balance of minerals I experience no cravings and Himalayan rock salt contains a lot of minerals and trace elements.

*** USEFUL FACT *** *Balancing the 'mineral wheel' is based on decades of science and one that any farmer could elaborate on from their experience with soil science. Get it right, and a long healthy life most likely awaits you. Get it wrong and it is simply a matter of time until a symptom appears ... See NOTES.*

Himalayan crystal rock salt contains 84 of the 92 known minerals and trace elements, which are identical to those in the human body and therefore are easily absorbed and assimilated. A spoonful of this vibrant liquid is added to all my filtered water drinks and cooked vegetables.

If your local health food store does not sell Himalayan

rock salt, then you'll be able to find suppliers on IHERB as well as Ebay.

*** **USEFUL FACT** *** *Make salt brine (sole) by filling a glass jar about 1/4 of the way with Himalayan salt. Fill the rest of the way with filtered water. Add a plastic lid (not metal!). Keep refilling your jar with salt and water when it runs low. It lasts indefinitely. See NOTES.*

Nowadays, I only ever have my drinks on the rocks, and Himalayan rocks at that.

AFTERWORD
PLEASE DON'T
FOLLOW MY DIET.

Please don't follow my diet. Why would I give you my diet and then ask you not to follow it? Why would I call the diet a well-balanced restricted diet perfect for all kinds of conditions and then ask readers to not copy it?

Because I don't want anyone to be writing me saying that they followed my diet and it did not work for him or her. I don't know any of my readers, so how could I possibly be designing a diet for any of them? Apart from not knowing any of my readers, I am not a dietitian, nor am I medically qualified. I completed a course on psychotherapy once and I did a number of medical practice management courses. Over the years, I've had an interest in healing and I haphazardly studied religion, health, and naturopathy, in that order. None of my studies qualify me to professionally design diets for others.

I know from managing medical clinics and being married to a doctor that before treating any conditions, such as, for instance, acne, mood swings, and the like, a person should have a chat with their preferred health professional and make sure that no easily treatable or serious conditions are overlooked.

The diet I devised is for me. My readers will have to come up with their own diet plan. I'm sharing my diet with my readers because it may give other people who suffer from food intolerances, for whatever reasons, some ideas of what to organise for themselves and their family with the help of their own health practitioners for their own specific conditions.

My diet may be quite restricted, yet it contains the basic nutrients that a human body needs to function, such as water, protein, carbohydrates, oils, vitamins, minerals, amino acids, and so on. I lived on this diet for five solid years. Nothing else. It worked for me!

Thanks to this diet, which took a load off my digestive system, I've progressed quite a bit and at present I am following directions of a number of health professionals, including Greg Turner, as well as dietary guidelines from Dr Wilson. I have added in to this book my adaption of his dietary guidelines as a bonus recovery diet after this Afterword. I'll probably be following this diet for quite some years to come, because even though this diet is simple, it is very comprehensive and based on sound scientific evidence.

I have been extremely fortunate to have met with outstanding medical and health practitioners who've helped and still are helping me on my way. Some of these people are listed on the *Thank You* page as my favourite people.

I credit my Creator with my progress and health and I wish for all of my readers' abundant and excellent health in wonderful company, and to never want for any.

BONUS DIET
OSFA (2)

UPDATE

I started writing this book in the year 2013 and it is now near the end of the year 2015. I have discovered a few new things since writing this book. One is that I appear to have some dodgy shock absorbers in my back, and I'll keep you posted on how these will be healed. Secondly, I discovered that I need to take B vitamins for my nervous system, and I noticed quite a bit of improvement since doing this. Thirdly, I discovered that I can eat many more items than I thought I was able to, as long as whatever I eat is organic! For years, I wasn't able to tolerate broccoli or spinach or kale or quinoa or rice, but I can now have these foods in small amounts ... as long as they are organic. The same applies with eggs and onions.

This discovery filled me with fresh hope and renewed vigour to follow Dr Wilson's diet suggestions. Following is my adaptation of his suggestions, and I feel better and more energetic on this diet. I am still relatively immobile, but my mustard seed of faith has been planted and carefully watered whilst steadily growing into a big tree. Climbing that tree will be my next victory.

I've made a few discoveries about my belief system and how this has affected my health. I want to share this because it is quite extraordinary how seemingly innocent thoughts can manifest quite powerfully in one's life.

When I worked all hours in our clinics there were many

times where I was so utterly exhausted that I would mutter under my breath, 'It will take me years to recover from this, it will take me years to get over this.' And guess what? It has been well over a decade of literally 'just laying around,' because that's all I've been able to manage.

Thoughts and words are extremely powerful. Use them wisely.

> *"Watch your thoughts, for they become words.*
> *Watch your words, for they become actions.*
> *Watch your actions, for they become habits.*
> *Watch your habits, for they become character.*
> *Watch your character, for it becomes your destiny."*

The next step

After about five years, I've stopped drinking the salty water. It served me well for the years that I did, but it is now time to give it a rest and start drinking more greens in an attempt to get a larger range of the minerals and vitamins I need.

The next diet I call the recovery OSFA (2) diet plan because this is my next step, step two. I believe that this diet also qualifies as a One Size Fits All diet.

One of the big discoveries in the process of transferring onto this diet was that I can eat many more items than I could previously, as long as they are organic.
Dr Wilson advocates that the abundance of minerals found in the large quantity of greens and root vegetables in his diet is what aids the rebuilding and healing of the body.

OSFA (2) BONUS
RECOVERY DIET

Breakfast

- · 1 slice of buttered gluten-free toast
- · egg, cheese, avocado or sardines as topping
- · quarter of an apple

Lunch

- · 80% Boiled vegetables/herbs (minerals/vitamins)
- · 10% quinoa or rice (carbohydrates)
- · 10% egg, tofu, sardines, kippers or chicken (protein)
- · Quarter of an apple or sauerkraut (for digestion)

Dinner

- · Cup of thick blended vegetable soup
- · Small dollop of sour cream
- · Few blue corn chips on the side
- · Quarter of an apple

Drinks

Drink only one hour before or after meals
- . One spoonful of mixed greens in a large glass of warm water in the morning
- . Camomile tea at night
- . Throughout the day 3 litres of mineral or filtered water on its own or together with ½ spoonful of wheat-grass powder or a homemade green juice.

The above are every day meals. Once more, this is all I eat

nowadays, nothing else whatsoever other than what is listed on these pages. All ingredients are organic. I am not able to tolerate anything non-organic.

Breakfast

It is nice to have toast topped with cheese, and when I have sardines, to add smidgen of mustard for extra nutrients and flavour.

Lunch

Every day the boiled vegetables consist of 30% cruciferous, 30% root and 30% leafy greens with 10% herbs.

On hot days my daughter wraps the precooked vegetables, cold from the fridge, in a sheet of nori and/or a rice wrap with a topping of tahini and the protein stuffed inside.

Dinner

When the temperature is above 25 degrees Celcius we may decide to have the soup for dinner cold.

When I share with others, they may have lentils or meat balls in their soup and a toasted slice of buttered French stick with cheese. There are people who sprinkle hemp seeds on their soup for protein, but this is considered illegal in Australia.

Delicious

What is so delicious about my bonus recovery diet is the addition of plentiful herbs and spices as mentioned below. I was not able to eat spices and herbs, other than salt, when I was eating my more limited diet. This was because at the time I either was not able to tolerate herbs and spices, or I was not aware that I could have many more food items, as long as they were organic.

What my daughter finds so delicious about my diet nowadays is that she only has to cook a few times during the week.

It takes her around five minutes to chop up the vegetables for the thick vegetable soup; add twenty minutes for the soup maker, and this produces around five serves which keeps good in the fridge for two to three days.

To chop up and boil the vegetables and herbs for the clear vegetable soup takes around half an hour all up. This soup also gets stored in the fridge for 3 days and some of this clear vegetable soup gets frozen for when the organic supply is low.

She soaks quinoa and rice overnight and after this it takes around twenty minutes to simmer with the vegetables, herbs and spices. She makes plenty of this also and stores the surplus in the fridge for up to three days.

By following the above routine my daughter only has to prepare breakfast every day which takes around fifteen minutes and my lunches and dinners are, more often than not, pre-prepared and only need heating up.

I am looking forward to add in fresh home-grown sprouts

such as sunflower and broccoli sprouts but we haven't been successful with this as yet. We're looking at ways to deal with the mould/fungi which can be a problem in subtropical climates.

Overall I find organic produce tastier than the mass produced varieties and the addition of spices, herbs and sauces ensures that each and every meal of my recovery diet is delicious!

INGREDIENTS IN DETAIL FOR THE
OSFA (2) BONUS RECOVERY DIET

Just to give my readers a bit of an idea about the vegetables that are cooked up for me every day, I have included a list below. At this stage I cannot source or tolerate all of them as yet, and an organic garden is on top of my wish list.

Every day the boiled vegetables consist of 30% cruciferous, 30% root and 30% leafy greens with 10% herbs.

My diet consists of around 80% of boiled vegetables and 10% protein and 10% carbohydrates.

According to Dr Wilson, the OSFA2 diet (this is my label, not his, and contains my adaptation of his guidelines) is extremely alkaline-forming. And as I understand it, a mix of the items as mentioned below, combined with adequate protein such as fish, meat, dairy, chicken, lentils, eggs as well as carbohydrates such as rice, bread, quinoa, pasta takes care of all our nutritional needs. If you can tolerate this, add a dash of cold pressed virgin olive or coconut oil.

Cruciferous vegetables

Any combination of vegetables in season: broccoli, brussels sprouts, onion, garlic, cauliflower, and any colour cabbage.

Root vegetables

Any combination of sweet potato, carrot, swedes, turnips, beetroot and also pumpkin of any kind.

Leafy greens

Any combination of spinach, silver beet, coloured chard, various kinds of kale, bok choy, and other varieties of Asian greens. Also nasturtium leaves as well as flowers and rocket. We add green beans to this mix also.

Herbs

Basil, coriander, oregano, lovage, continental parsley, thyme, rosemary, and mint.

Spices

Sea salt, ginger, kelp, tumeric, cayenne pepper, and garlic.

Sauces and condiments

Hummus, tahini, tamari, miso paste, guacamole, and mustard.

WEEKLY MENU

Monday – Wednesday – Friday

Breakfast: gluten-free toast with organic butter and lactose-free cheese and/or egg, piece of apple.

Lunch: clear vegetable soup created from greens such as rainbow chard, silver beet and herbs, celery and garlic, onion, ginger, dried shitake mushrooms, and gluten-free noodles.

Dinner: thick vegetable soup created from root vegetables such as carrots, beetroot, and also pumpkin, green beans with small dollop of sour cream, a few purple corn chips, and apple on the side.

Tuesday – Thursday – Saturday

Breakfast: gluten-free toast with organic butter and sardines and/or egg, piece of apple.

Lunch: small portion of very well cooked rice or quinoa with green leafy vegetables and herbs and strips of organic fried eggs, boiled chicken, or small amount of sardines or kippers.

Dinner: thick vegetable soup created from root vegetables such as pumpkin, carrots, beetroot and green beans with small dollop of sour cream, a few purple corn chips and apple on the side.

Sunday

Breakfast: gluten-free toast with organic butter and soft-boiled organic egg, piece of apple.

Lunch: clear vegetable soup created from spinach greens and herbs, celery and garlic, onion, ginger, dried shitake mushrooms, and gluten-free noodles and a few bits of chicken.

Dinner: thick vegetable soup created from root vegetables such as pumpkin, carrots, beetroot, and green beans with small dollop of sour cream, a few purple corn chips, and apple on the side.

Drinks

One tablespoon of juiced carrot and greens and herbs such as spinach, kale, celery, parsley, coriander, garlic, onion, ginger, and lemon in a large glass of warm water. This stays good in the fridge for three days and I have this throughout the day, but not after lunch,
Other than that, I only drink herbal teas and filtered water.

Snacks

If I get hungry between meals I usually have a mug of clear vegetable or miso soup, and occasionally a bit of 1/3 banana or apple or pawpaw with a little yoghurt. Maybe one brazil nut or a couple of almonds. Every now and then I'll have a quarter of a coconut macaroon or half a handful of purple corn chips or Irish moss herb cooked in water and set in the fridge with some cream. Once in a blue moon I can have a tiny bit of chocolate. Yeah! Eating regular chocolate is linked with longevity and I am in training.

TWO DIETS
INSTEAD OF ONE

ONE BONUS DIET

Two Diets Instead of One

I don't mean to confuse anyone by giving out two diets instead of one. The second diet, the bonus one called the OSFA (2) Recovery Diet, is what I am on now in 2015. The OSFA (2) diet is a progression from the previous, quite strict, low reactive elimination diet. Five, six years ago, I would not have been able to tolerate the OSFA (2) diet. I am convinced however, that the OSFA (2) diet is by far the better choice over the long term.

This book has been around two years in the making, and even though I could expand on this book or even start a whole new book on my progress and diet, I would prefer to get this book out quickly. I know that many people with dietary problems, for whatever reasons, will benefit from hearing my story because it will enable and encourage them to come up with their own version suited to their own unique situation.

We know how hard it is when most food substances bring on severe reactions, and no matter where we looked, we weren't able to find an affordable diet which worked for me.

My kids and I literally spent years trying to figure out what works and what doesn't, and the diet I have been on for five years works for anyone with food intolerances, such as dairy (substitute with lactose free, kefir or coconut yoghurt), gluten, meat, sugar, fructose, grains, flours, nuts, seeds, eggs, beans, soy, and lentils.

We were completely at our wits' end as to what I should eat because I was not able to eat anything at all without massive negative reactions. It was only through prayer and trial and error that we finally managed to come up with the diet, which I've now been on for five solid years.

It was through the suggestion of a good friend that I discovered that I can now tolerate more foods than I thought I was able to, as long as these foods have been organically grown. I seem to have developed a huge reaction to pesticides used on ordinary foods.

Adding in regular vitamin B supplements of the folate kind (not folic acid) also helped to increase my tolerance to certain foods and supplements.

I want to share this info with anyone else who is stressing about their diet as soon as possible and not wait another year or so perfecting and updating the information that is available to me today.

Links have been provided to all the fabulous health practitioners who have helped and are still helping me on my way. It has taken me more than a decade to compile this list. Many of these outstanding practitioners will consult by phone, which is a wonderful thing for people who are confined to bed and in need of medical assistance. I love and embrace them all.

Obviously there is much more to my story of survival than just the diet. The spine plays an important role also.

Impingements will affect your nervous system and restrict the flow of nutrients. Emotional upheavals are to be avoided at all costs, and so on.

It's just that I hear and read about so many people suffering because of their diet that I'm keen to share what worked for me as soon as possible at least with regards to diet.

PS.
Did I mention my gallbladder attacks? I don't think I did. I've licked them, kinda. I want to share with you how. Contact me at www.mosaichouse.co/contact-us and I'll let you know how I seem to have both my pancreatic as well as gallbladder attacks mostly under control now. Cause if I keep going here, this book will never finish.

MANY THANKS

To FAVOURITE PEOPLE AND FABULOUS WEBSITES

Dr Mark Donohoe at
www.mimpractice.com/doctors/#/drmark
Dr Andrew Ladhams at
www.barebonesmedicineco.com.au
Dr Deed at http://blogs.abc.net.au/files/khd--dr-gary-deed.mp3
Jim Golick at
www.naturescornucopia.com/nutritionalcounseling.html
Naturopath Grace at www.thenaturalfoodstore.com.au
Noel Batten at www.noelbatten.com
Dr Alex Goodheart at www.beachsidechiropractic.com.au
Dr Viv Taylor at www.ibukihealth.com
Dr Emerson at www.drgregemerson.com
Meir Schneider at www.self-healing.org/meir-schneider
Celine at www.frogshop.com.au
Mark at www.gonaturalfoods.com.au
Dr John Christopher at www.herballegacy.com
Dr Lawrence Wilson at
www.drlwilson.com/ARTICLES/VEG DIET.htm
Dr Todd Lizon at www.lifestyleintegration.com.au
Dr Ben Kim at www.drbenkim.com
Kimberley Geswein at www.kimberlygeswein.com
Jonathan Feinberg at www.mrfeinberg.com
Leslie Taylor at www.rain-tree.com
The iherb team at www.iherb.com
The Mosaic House team at www.mosaichouse.co

MORE FAVOURITE PEOPLE

My hero Herbalist Greg Turner

Our friend Michael

Dr Mutti Kahn
Physio Mark
Homeopath Lindsay Smith
Acupuncturist Aihua Bei
Osteopath Jane Little
Remedial Masseuse
Glynis Orr
Dietician Peter St Henry

My writing buddies Robyn, Kathi, Colleen and Ian
My fabulous editor Elaine

Colleen, Ann, Claudia, Jude, Jan, Lainey
siblings Monica and Maria.
My children

MY FAVOURITE COMMUNITY

I've been out of action for more than a decade and it has taken me at least a couple of years to write this book. After this I did not really know how to get my book out into the world. I am not in a position to send endless letters to book publishing companies or invest a huge amount and have other people publish my book for me. I was more than a little annoyed by my situation because I know that there are people out there who will benefit from reading my book.

I did not really know where to go from having a pdf of my book to having my book successfully published on Amazon till I came across a post called 'Self-publishing Success Summit.' The promise of this summit was that I would receive a blueprint how to go from "no idea" to bestselling author in 3 steps and this included a free video course which reveals how to write, publish, and market your first book, even if you don't have time, writing skills, or a book idea.

I already had a book but did not really know how to get it out into the world. I found Chandler Bolt's insider knowledge fascinating because he shares this so freely. His enthusiasm is infectious, and I decided to sign up and see where it would take me.

This is a MASSIVE THANK YOU!!! to the wonderful community of Self-Publishing School which supports and helps Indie authors to write their books and publish them. I do not know if without their help I would have been able to get my book published on Amazon as it is right now. I am tremendously grateful for not only the expertise and know-how offered, but in particular the step-by-step guidance and enormous back-up support and warm and inviting community. I truly believe that this kind of support and community is unequalled in the book publishing industry.

You know how you can be a member of face book groups and no-one ever notices your posts? Well not with this private group. They truly are one of a kind and I plan to be part of their group for a long time to come. Chandler Bolt who is the brain child of SPS is only a young kid but one smart cookie! All kudos to you Chandler, and your team!

If you want to check out what these guys are all about and join me as part of this caring and supportive community you can visit www.mosaichouse.co/my-story-of-survival and sign up for the free video course or Summit or all that's on offer.

NOTES

LOW FODMAP DIET

Dr Sue Shepherd has proven, through her pioneering PhD research, that limiting dietary FODMAPs is an effective treatment for people with symptoms of IBS. The low FODMAP diet has been published in international medical journals and is now accepted and recommended as one of the most effective dietary therapies for IBS. http://shepherdworks.com.au/disease-information/low-fodmap-diet.

INCREASE LIFESPAN

The CALERIE study is being carried out at the Pennington Biomedical Research Center (Baton Rouge, Louisiana), the Jean Mayer USDA Human Nutrition Research Center on Aging at Tufts University (Boston, Massachusetts) and the Washington University School of Medicine (St. Louis, Missouri).[1] It is hoped that caloric restriction reduces the incidence of cardiovascular disease and cancer and leads to a longer life, as has been demonstrated previously in numerous animal studies. http://calerie.dcri.duke.edu/

STRESS AFFECTS GUT HEALTH

Chronic stress (and other negative emotions like anger, anxiety and sadness) can trigger symptoms and full-blown disease in your gut. As Harvard researchers explain:

"Psychology combines with physical factors to cause pain and other bowel symptoms. Psychosocial factors influence the actual physiology of the gut, as well as symptoms. In other words, stress (or depression or other psychological factors) can affect movement and contractions of the GI

tract, cause inflammation, or make you more susceptible to infection.
http://articles.mercola.com/sites/articles/archive/2012/04/0
9/chronic-stress-gut-effects.aspx

DRUGS AFFECT GUT HEALTH

Simply put, antibiotics are poisons that are used to kill and likely help fungi to proliferate within the human body. Treatment with antibiotics can cause irreversible changes in the gut.
http://www.sciencedaily.com/releases/2013/01/130109081
145.htm
http://articles.mercola.com/sites/articles/archive/2003/06/1
8/antibiotics-bacteria.aspx

FOOD INTOLERANCES AND ALLERGIES

A food intolerance is he inability to fully digest a food. When your body cannot completely process a food - the result is partially digested proteins and sugars. This happens especially with foods like grains, milk and sugars. Protein breakdown fragments in particular cause trouble because the body does not recognise them as 'friendly'. This sets up inflammation and disrupts bodily functions. . . causing dozens of symptoms and can develop into disease if left unattended. https://www.foodintol.com/food-sensitivities

CHRONIC STRESS

Chronic stress can trigger symptoms and full-blown disease in your gut and contribute to conditions such as Lupus, Chronic Fatigue Syndrome, Fibromyalgia, Myalgic Encephalomyelitis and Inflammatory bowel diseases and the like. As Harvard researchers explain: *"Stress (or depression or other psychological factors) can affect movement and contractions of the GI tract, cause inflammation, or make you more susceptible to infection."* http://articles.mercola.com/sites/articles/archive/2012/04/09/chronic-stress-gut-effects.aspx

RICE FACTS

Nearly half the world's 6.6 billion population eat rice as part of their staple diet and demand is expected to grow by 50 per cent by 2030. There are more than 40,000 varieties of rice. Rice is naturally gluten-free and low in fat. It contains all eight essential amino acids, folic acid, and is very low in sodium and cholesterol.
http://www.tilda.com/us/rice-facts
http://www.tilda.com/our-rice/why-basmati-is-best
\

ELIMINATION DIET

An elimination diet is a diet devised to identify foods that an individual cannot consume without adverse effects. An elimination diet can also be used temporarily to ease the burden on a challenged digestive system. Start off with a diet as basic as you can manage and then slowly introduce new ingredients. A good rule of thumb is to introduce one new ingredient every three to four days. It is also a good idea, whenever possible, to rotate the menu and not eat the same ingredient day after day.

DIGESTIVE ENZYMES

Digestive enzymes are substances produced by our bodies that help us to digest the foods we eat. These enzymes are secreted by the various parts of our digestive system and

they help to break down food components such as proteins, carbohydrates, and fats. As we age and due to illness, the ability to produce these enzymes decreases and we may have to supplement our diet with enzymes to be able to properly absorb our food. I prefer NOW Optimal Digestive and NOW Dairy Digest.
http://au.iherb.com/search?kw=now+enzymes&sug=co+en zymes#p=1

FABULOUS NATURAL SUPPLEMENTS
Enter code MIN221 for a five or ten dollar discount with your first order at www.Iherb.com.

GOLDENSEAL
Goldenseal's ability as a "natural antibiotic" has given this herb a great reputation in the herbal lore. Digestive secretions in the stomach are increased by taking the remedies made from the goldenseal. The remedy also has an astringent action on the mucous membranes lining the gut; this checks the spread of inflammation in the area at the same time. Do not use for prolonged period of time.
http://www.herbs2000.com/herbs/herbs_goldenseal.htm

REACTIONS TO ANTIBIOTICS
Side effects, allergies and reactions to antibiotics are not that unusual. Common side effects are rashes, diarrhea, abdominal pain, nausea/vomiting, hypersensitivity, dizziness.
http://www.drugs.com/article/antibiotic-sideeffects-allergies-reactions.html

OSFA DIET

Stands for One Size Fits All diet because virtually anyone would be able to tolerate the diet I have been on for five years. And if someone is not able to tolerate some of the ingredients, then the diet can be easily adjusted by replacing these ingredients with some of the examples mentioned in the book. The low reactive OSFA (1) is my ten-ingredient-only diet and OSFA (2) is the recovery diet which is based on suggestions made by Dr Wilson and all good nutritionists and dietitians.

MINERAL BALANCE

Balancing the 'mineral wheel' is based on decades of science and one that any farmer could elaborate on from their experience with soil science. Get it right, and a long healthy life most likely awaits you. Get it wrong and it is simply a matter of time until a symptom appears.
http://www.lifestyleintegration.com.au/learning-centre/articles/32-balancing-the-mineral-wheel.html

LOW BLOOD VOLUME

Visit http://phoenixrising.me/archives/11814 for more on living with low blood volume by Dr David Bell.

COELIAC GENE

People who have been diagnosed as a coeliac appear to have a particular gene. High-risk genetic patterns recognised for coeliac disease and gluten sensitivity are DQ2 and DQ8.

ALTERNATIVES TO ANTIBIOTICS
Garlic is a great alternative, if tolerated, as are certain herbal combinations, which need to be taken for prolonged periods of time to be effective. Check out www.rain-tree.com for the best natural medicine I've come across.

SCURVY
Scurvy in an otherwise well young man, the Medical Journal of Australia.
www.mja.com.au/journal/2006/185/6/scurvy-otherwise-well-young-man

POTATO ONLY DIET
I ate 20 Potatoes a day, for 60 days straight! Visit
http://20potatoesaday.com

ACUTE PANCREATITIS TIAL
Dutch trial of probiotics in acute pancreatitis is to be investigated after deaths (24) by Tjaard U Hoogenraad, retired neurologist from the University of Utrecht in Holland 10th April 2013 (-edit July 2015 this link does not appear active at the moment-).
www.bmj.com/content/336/7639/296.3/rr/640208.

ANN WIGMORE STORY
Ann Wigmore's story on the benefits of wheatgrass can be downloaded for free from
http://loveforlife.com.au/files/whysuffer.pdf

WHEATGRASS

Wheatgrass is a good source of Protein and Potassium, and a very good source of Dietary Fibre, Vitamin A, Vitamin C, Vitamin E (Alpha Tocopherol), Vitamin K, Thiamin, Riboflavin, Niacin, Vitamin B6, Pantothenic Acid, Iron, Zinc, Copper, Manganese and Selenium.
http://nutritiondata.self.com/facts/custom/900675/2#ixzz3sD9rfwXL

PRAYER VERSES AND SCRIPTURAL REFERENCES

'Oh Sing unto the Lord' from Psalm 96:1
'When the singers were as one' from 2 Chronicles 5:13-14
'His merciful kindness is great towards us' from Psalm 117
'By the Word of the Lord were the heavens made' from Psalm 33:6-9
'Please forsake not the work of thine own hands' from Psalm 138:8
'God's Word shall not return void' from Isaiah 55:11
'We waited patiently for the Lord' from Psalm 40:1-3
'We walk with God like Enoch did' from Genesis 5:24, Matthew 6:10

ABOUT SALINE AND HIMALAYAN ROCK SALT

Saline solution for intravenous infusion consists of 0.90% w/v of NaCl, about 300 mOsm/L or 9.0 g per liter. 9 grams NaCl is equal to around 1.62 level teaspoons of sodium chloride or salt in a litre of water. Himalayan rock salt is about the best possible quality of salt available. To create a brine, add rocks (salt) to a covered glass jar and fill with water, let sit for a day, and add a spoonful of this brine at a time to a glass of water or two at a time to a cooking pot filled with vegetables.

http://empoweredsustenance.com/himalayan-salt-benefits/

DR BELL RESEARCH
More on Dr David Bell's research on intravenous fluid as a treatment for me/cfs and orthostatic intolerance used to be on www.drdavidsbell.com. He mentioned severe risk of infection at a rate of 20% per line per year, which requires antibiotic treatment. Infection is due to the indwelling catheter. (-edit July 2015 this link does not appear active at the moment-).

PROMISING RESEARCH
Brad Crouch, Medical Reporter for the *Adelaide Advertiser,* published an article on 16th October, 2015 about promising research with regards to peanut allergy breakthrough. Brad reports that The Flinders Medical Centre project by paediatric allergist Dr Billy Tao uses a two-step technique, initially boiling peanuts for two hours to make them less allergenic. Children are fed these peanuts to partially desensitise them, then when they show no signs of allergic reaction, the children are fed roasted peanuts to further increase their tolerance. Of 14 participants aged under 16 who all had serious allergic reactions, 10 have completed the first stage and are now eating roasted peanuts daily, while four continue to eat boiled peanuts daily.
I mention this research here because I belief this technique potentially holds many promises for overcoming other allergies too.

KOSHER FISH

Sardines, kippers, whiting, and anchovies are my favourites. Some say that salmon, tuna, herring, and mackerel are also kosher, but I am not sure about this because various fishermen I know give conflicting reports about these fish having scales or not. Maybe this depends on the area, I don't know. Pregnant women are cautioned not to eat much tuna due to the mercury content.

HOME MADE AND HOME GROWN

Whenever possible, make at home the yoghurt and kefir and sauerkraut and grow your own organic vegetables and sprouts. It is not that hard to do and the benefits as well as the savings are great.

THANK YOU!!

Visit

If you have any questions at all, or just to say hi you can visit me and share your thoughts and questions with me at www.mosaichouse.co.

I really like to hear from you and am happy to share whatever worked for me.

Share

Please share this book with anyone that you think may benefit from it. There are many people nowadays who suffer from gut problems and food intolerances, chemical sensitivities and allergies. If just one person benefits from reading this book, it was worth writing.

Third Edition

The second edition of this book was a leaner copy and made available for free. However this meant that I could not have the book published on Amazon and this prompted my decision to bring out a third edition (the one you are reading now), which includes more of my testimony, the Scripture verses which got me prompt attention at Emergency Intake, and the one-page weekly recovery diet which I currently use.

Thank you very much!

Book reviews are really important because they help customers find the book they're after. As an author your review helps me make the next book better. If you did not enjoy the book, thank you for contacting me and letting me know how I can improve the next edition. And if you enjoyed the book thank you for leaving a review and tell others about it!

Thank you for your support!

Mimi

Following is an easy shopping list to purchase healthy, tasty and nutritious food to prepare delicious meals as well as a food elimination guide and a 'Benefits of Stress Infographic.'

EASY SHOPPING LIST TO PURCHASE

HEALTHY, TASTY, AND NUTRITIOUS FOOD TO PREPARE DELICIOUS MEALS.

Daily boiled vegetables of 30% cruciferous, 30% root, and 30% leafy greens, with 10% herbs.

My diet consists of around 80% boiled vegetables and 10% protein and 10% carbohydrates.

PROTEIN

Fish such as sardines, salmon, kippers, anchovies or mackerel, organic meat, lactose-free cheese, chicken, lentils, beans, eggs, and tofu. (I don't eat tofu, lentils, beans, or meat myself)

CARBODYDRATES

Organic rice, quinoa and gluten-free bread and pasta such as rice noodles.

FATS

Organic butter, cold-pressed organic virgin olive or coconut oil, and sour cream.

CRUCIFEROUS VEGETABLES

Any combination of vegetables in season: broccoli, Brussels sprouts, onion, garlic, cauliflower, and any colour cabbage.

ROOT VEGETABLES

Any combination of root vegetables in season such as sweet potato, carrot, swedes, turnips, beetroot and also pumpkin of any kind.

LEAFY GREENS

Any combination of whatever is in season such as spinach, silver beet, coloured chard, various kinds of kale, bokchoy, and other varieties of Asian greens. Also nasturtium leaves as well as flowers and rocket. We add green beans, fennel, and celery to this mix also.

HERBS

Basil, coriander, oregano, lovage, continental parsley, thyme, rosemary, and mint.

SPICES

Sea salt, ginger, kelp, turmeric, cayenne pepper, and garlic.

SAUCES AND CONDIMENTS

Hummus, tahini, tamari, miso paste, guacamole, and mustard.

OTHER

Organic apples, lemon, pawpaw, purple chips, miso, herbal teas, dried shitake mushrooms, figs, and once in a blue moon we get nuts and bananas.

ELMINATION DIET

WHY GO ON AN ELIMINATION DIET?

There are many different reasons ranging from severe health problems to experiencing slight discomfort after eating certain foods. Usually people go on elimination diet to figure out why their health is declining or why their digestive system is upset.

Before you consider going on an elimination diet.

When your health is declining and/or your digestive system is upset, PLEASE go see a doctor and have him check you out and follow the doctor's advice. If you do not get the results you're after get a referral to a dietician and/or visit a nutritionist or a naturopath. Only consider going on an elimination diet after this. There could be all different kinds of reasons why you're not feeling on top of the world, and you owe it to yourself to see a qualified medical health practitioner to help you get to the bottom of this.

How does one go on an elimination diet?

Take it easy. If you expect too much, you're likely to fail. In our clinics, people were told to only eat brown or white rice for 3 days, as much as they liked, but nothing else aside from the rice, other than water. Then slowly add back in the various food groups one at a time to see if they were tolerated. Needless to say that many people failed because they simply weren't able to eat food as bland as that.

If you are able to do this, I would say give it a go, because this is the quickest way you're likely to find out what foods cause you trouble. I wasn't able to do this because I couldn't tolerate rice either.

What is not allowed?

Okay, you're going to hate me saying this, but chances are that the food you like the most and find the hardest to give up is the food that gives you the most grief. Sorry, but you asked. That just seems to be the way it works. After a period of time our system tends to become sensitive to our favourite foods. I used to LOVE a little chocolate mousse, which I bought from our local supermarket. One day, bam! Even a few tiny spoonfuls gave me a massive migraine. Did they put different additives in the mousse? Unlikely, because my daughters could still eat the same product, without any trouble.

If you are not able to let go of your favourite foods for a while you are unlikely to discover what is upsetting your gut. All through my childhood I suffered from a sore tummy after meals. It wasn't till I left home that this stopped. I also stopped having yogurt at the same time.

All through my childhood I suffered from sinus problems. After I left home I stopped eating dairy, and for the first time my nostrils sucked in fresh air. Nowadays I can have minimal (organic and/or lactose free) amounts as long as I take digestive enzymes with it.

The main culprits for most people usually are dairy, eggs, soy, gluten, fast foods, alcohol, coffee, and sugary flavoured and processed foods. Most of the things that you normally eat or drink are suspects unless this is organic, fresh, and unprocessed. The less processed the food, the less stress is caused to any of your organs.

All your favourites, such as ice creams, cookies, chocolate, coffee, and so on are potentially problematic. Usually the foods which are the hardest to let go of are the more processed foods. I've never heard anyone say that they cannot live one day without their broccoli. If you buy tins, and packaged foods, and I suggest that you don't, but if you do buy tins look for those without additives such as salt and sugar and colours and flavours.

In my case, I could not tolerate any sugar either, no flours of any kind, no beans, no seeds, no nuts. I couldn't eat meat (too hard to digest), and even fresh fish straight from the fishery caused me grief. Tofu didn't work for me, nor did dairy or cheeses.
I wasn't able to eat onion or garlic, none of the sulphurous foods that everyone raves about these days such as broccoli, cabbage, kale, Brussels sprouts. All of these would give me massive cramps and bloating to the point where it became extremely painful and unbearable.

Google may well be your best friend, and there are some very well-though-out elimination charts on the Web from reputable sources. If you were to be as brazen as try my suggestions, this will be entirely AT YOUR OWN RISK!! Because it worked for me does not mean that it will work for you; I am not medically qualified!!

What is allowed on my elimination diet?

Vegetable soups are allowed. But I would not add potato or tomato or capsicum or beans or zucchini or kale to the soup. Only if you know 100% for sure that these foods cause no problem would I add them to the soup.

Vegetable soups are a good idea because they will give you the minerals you need in an easily digestible format, as well as the fibre we need to be able to process food. Throughout the day you can have a light vegetable soup, as much as you like, hot or cold, with for instance, shredded spinach, green beans, parsley, coriander, gluten-free noodles, dried shitake mushrooms, and a little miso for flavour. At night you can have a soup made of root vegetables such as carrot and beetroot or sweet potato, and maybe pumpkin.

You can drink filtered water, green juices, herbal teas, and eat meat that comes from organic grass-fed cows, organic eggs, and fish. Eggs are known to cause problems, but organic eggs often can be tolerated. For this reason it's best to start without eggs and add them in later.

So what to do?

Consider the rice-only diet. If you cannot hack that, consider my ten-ingredient-only diet (read My Story of Survival) or the vegetable soups.

First see a doctor, please.

The main thing to consider when your gut is upset is first of all see a doctor and have him check you over to make sure that there is nothing really sinister going on. Then follow up on your doctor's advice. If you get no joy out of this I would recommend you see a dietician, nutritionist and or a naturopath.

If you still, despite following their recommendations, are not improving, you can consider my suggestions. They worked for me after trial and error after I experienced problems with my gut, my heart, my appendix, gallbladder, and pancreas.

I found that for a number of years I had to cut out all fats and oils because my pancreas was not able to tolerate any. My gallbladder would get upset with minty things such as herbal mint teas and so on. My heart would burn after fatty foods. Trial and error led me to the diet that worked for me. But everyone is unique with their own unique problems and, other than for a short period only, I honestly don't think that it is a good idea to live on ten-ingredients-only. It worked for me, but my situation is rather unique.

After years we made the wonderful discovery that eating a little apple with my meals kept my digestive processes happy. This combined with having digestive enzymes with the meals and the occasional spoonful of vinegar in a glass of water helped hugely towards being able to eat meals without upsets.

Remove all hindrances

The main thing is to remove all hindrances and aggravating factors. This means that you should aim to remove, as much as possible, whatever it is that is upsetting your gut. This can be emotional upsets, environmental, physical, mental, food items, or perhaps even look at the water you drink.

Once the aggravating factors are removed, you need to heal whatever was damaged by providing soothing and healing circumstances, environmental, physical, emotional, mental, and food.

After this you can start to provide nourishing and building blocks to build up the immune system and get back to being in a position of good health.

1. Remove hindrances
2. Heal what's damaged
3. Build up the system

Doctors and nutritionists and dieticians and naturopaths are trained to do exactly that, and they should be your first port of call.

Oodles of faith worked miracles

I firmly believe that my diet saved my life. I reckon that the oodles of faith, which were a main part of my diet, worked miracles. My wish and prayer for you is that you will find a diet which works for you and that will sustain and nourish you for many years to come.

'BENEFITS OF STRESS'

This infographic is courtesy of Robyn Spooner
author of the book 'Benefits of Stress'
Available from Amazon

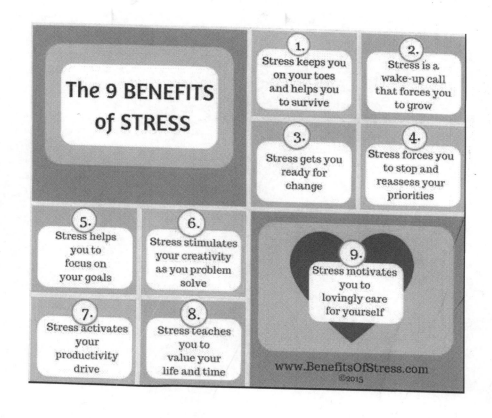

BOOKS BY MIMI EMMANUEL

www.amazon.com/author/mimiemmanuel

www.mimiemmanuel.com

My Story of Survival
Mimi's Book Launch Plan
God Healed Me
God Healed Me Prayer Journal
The Holy Grail of Book Launching

Anthologies contributed to:
Glimpses of Light
Like a Girl

Scripture Cards:
www.freescripturecards.com
www.mosaichouse.co

- Copyright myemmanuel 2015 -

28289413R00080

Made in the USA
San Bernardino, CA
06 March 2019